BWLS

BASIC WILDERNESS LIFE SUPPORT®

PREVENTION · DIAGNOSIS · TREATMENT · EVACUATION

A Text for Wilderness First Responder Courses

SENIOR EDITOR
RICHARD INGEBRETSEN, MD, PHD
CLINICAL INSTRUCTOR OF MEDICINE
UNIVERSITY OF UTAH SCHOOL OF MEDICINE

EDITORS
DAVID DELLA-GIUSTINA MD, FAWM
EMERGENCY MEDICINE RESIDENCY DIRECTOR
YALE UNIVERSITY SCHOOL OF MEDICINE

MATT SMITH MD, PHD
DIRECTOR, WILDERNESS MEDICINE OF UTAH
UNIVERSITY OF UTAH SCHOOL MEDICINE

Wilderness Medicine
University of Utah
School of Medicine

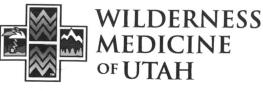

WILDERNESS MEDICINE OF UTAH

COPY EDIT
JULIE ROBERTS

COVER
DILLON JENSEN

ILLUSTRATIONS
MICHAEL DIDIER

RESEARCH
JUSTIN COLES

Edition 3.74 2013 by Travel Medicine Press

CONTRIBUTORS

P. Egan Anderson
Wilderness Medicine Program
University of Utah School of Medicine
Salt Lake City, Utah

Ali S. Arastu
Keck School of Medicine
University of Southern California
Los Angeles, California

E. Wayne Askew, Ph.D.
Professor and Director, Division of Nutrition
Faculty, Advanced Wilderness Life Support
University of Utah School of Medicine
Salt Lake City, Utah

Jerome Bidinger, JD, PhD
Faculty, Advanced Wilderness Life Support
Wilderness Medicine Attorney
Scottsdale, Arizona

Chris Bazzoli
Medical Student
Ohio State University College of Medicine
Columbus, Ohio

Nick Blickenstaff
Medical Student
Wilderness Medicine Program
University of Utah School of Medicine
Salt Lake City, Utah

Jane Bowman, MD
University of Utah School of Medicine
Western Gynecological Clinic
Salt Lake City, Utah

Justin Coles
Wilderness Medicine Program
University of Utah School of Medicine
Salt Lake City, Utah

Garrett Coman
Medical Student
Wilderness Medicine Program
University of Utah School of Medicine
Salt Lake City, Utah

Andrew Crockett, MD
Department of General Surgery
Ohio State University College of Medicine
Columbus, Ohio

Sarah Crockett MD
Department of Emergency Medicine
Ohio State University College of Medicine
Columbus, Ohio

David Della-Giustina, MD, FAWM
Emergency Medicine Residency Program Director,
Yale University School of Medicine
New Haven, Connecticut

Nelson Diamond
Medical Student
Duke University School of Medicine
Durham, North Carolina

J. Nicholas Francis, PhD
Wilderness Medicine Program
University of Utah Department of Biochemistry
Salt Lake City, Utah

Joey Fyans, MD
Department of Physical and Rehabilitation Medicine,
University of Utah School of Medicine
Salt Lake City, Utah

William Gochnour
Wilderness Medicine Program
University of Utah School of Medicine
Salt Lake City, Utah

Colin Grissom, MD
Assistant Professor of Medicine
University of Utah School of Medicine
Co-Director, Shock Trauma ICU
Intermountain Regional Medical Center
President, Wilderness Medical Society
Salt Lake City, Utah

David Hile, MD
Department of Emergency Medicine
Madigan Army Medical Center
University of Washington
Tacoma, Washington

Richard J. Ingebretsen, MD, PhD
Professor, Department of Medical Physics
Adjunct Instructor, Department of Medicine
University of Utah School of Medicine
Medical Director Salt Lake County Sheriff Search and
Rescue
Salt Lake City, Utah

Nate Kofford, MD
Department of Anesthesia
Dartmouth Hitchcock Medical Center
Dartmouth University
Hanover, New Hampshire

Jackson Lever, MD
Department of Ophthalmology
William Beaumont University
Royal Oak, Michigan

R. William Mackie, MD
Associate Professor of Medicine
Department of Cardiology
University of Utah School of Medicine
Salt Lake City, Utah

Robert Quinn MD, FAAOS
Professor and Chairman
Orthopaedic Surgery
Residency Program Director
University of Texas Health Sciences
San Antonio, Texas

Jacob Radtke
Wilderness Medicine Program
University of Utah School of Medicine
Salt Lake City, Utah

Steven Roy NR-EMT FAWM
Medical Student
McGill University School of Medicine
Medical Advisor, Quebec Secours
Montreal, Quebec, Canada

Dean Tanner
Medical Student
University of Utah School of Medicine
Salt Lake City, Utah

Jason Tanner
Medical Student
University of Utah School of Medicine
Salt Lake City, Utah
Salt Lake County Sherriff Search and Rescue

James Tucker, PhD
Medical Student
University of Utah School of Medicine
Salt Lake City, Utah

Taylor Sandstrom
Wilderness Medicine Program
University of Utah School of Medicine
Salt Lake City, Utah

Paul Schmutz, DDS
Faculty, Advanced Wilderness Life Support
Wilderness Dentistry
Bountiful, Utah

Christian Smith
Medical Student
Ohio State University College of Medicine
Columbus, Ohio

Matt Smith, MD. PhD
University of Utah School of Medicine
Director, Wilderness Medicine of Utah
Salt Lake City, Utah

James Tucker
Medical Student
University of Utah School of Medicine
Salt Lake City, Utah

Ian Wedmore, MD
Department of Emergency Medicine,
Madigan Army Medical Center
University of Washington
Tacoma, Washington

Benjamin Woods, MD
University of Utah School of Mcdicine
Physician, Intermountain Health Care
Salt Lake City, Utah

G. Andrew Wright
Wilderness Medicine Program
University of Utah School of Medicine
Salt Lake City, Utah

Patrick Zimmerman
Medical Student
A.T. Still University
School of Osteopathic Medicine in Arizona
Mesa, Arizona

TABLE OF CONTENTS

INTRODUCTION
Wilderness Responders

Usually, travelers find themselves in the wilderness intentionally. The intrepid seek out unknown corners of the globe for recreation and adventure, and to experience the natural elements. The most beautiful and rugged places on earth are often the most distant from definitive medical care. While making great efforts to escape civilization, travelers simultaneously increase the chances of adverse outcomes, should a medical emergency present itself.

♦ DEFINITION ♦

Wilderness: Any place that is uncultivated, uninhabited, or inhabited only by wildlife.

Outdoor activities are increasing in popularity throughout the world. The wilderness offers adventurers a beautiful and challenging arena in which to hike, ski, run rivers, scuba dive, climb, bike, and so much more. However, injuries and illnesses are common in wilderness settings. Some diseases are even unique to the outdoors.

The excitement and increasing accessibility of outdoor activities attract large numbers of participants, many of whom have little or no backcountry, let alone wilderness, experience. Some of these people already have pre-existing medical conditions. Many bring more zeal than preparation and fitness to their chosen activity—thereby putting themselves distinctly at risk.

Because activities can take travelers to remote places, the responsibility for managing medical problems largely lies with the guides who take them there. A guide will doubtlessly encounter occasional medical problems and may be depended upon as an authority. The unique diseases of the wilderness—snakebites, high altitude cerebral edema, frostbite, lightning strike, and many others—are outside the scope of routine medicine. The skills and knowledge taught in first response medicine will provide you the knowledge and background to recognize and treat backcountry emergencies with confidence and will train you in prevention, diagnosis, treatment, and evacuation of backcountry injuries.

Wilderness medicine is a unique field of medicine. It incorporates aspects of:

- search & rescue
- physiology and pathophysiology
- clinical judgment and treatment
- creative improvisation
- psychology & group dynamics
- preventive medicine & public health

Wilderness medicine teaches about the body's response to extremes of the environment, such as cold, heat, altitude, and lack of water, and their attendant physical stresses. It also prepares wilderness first responders to anticipate the effects of these extremes on pre-existing medical conditions.

The hospital setting provides caregivers an environment that allows them to focus almost entirely on medical care. This is a luxury that is rarely afforded in the backcountry. The presence of fire, rain, cold, darkness, avalanche, rock fall, wind, treacherous rivers, or wild animals obviously complicates a situation. In such circumstances, heroism must be tempered by sensibility and the knowledge necessary to avoid creating additional victims. Even the most basic diagnostic equipment, such as a blood pressure cuff and stethoscope, may not be available in the wilderness. Learned skills, along with good judgment, must be honed in order to determine the severity of medical, surgical, and psychological emergencies. The BWLS® program offers evacuation guidelines for these situations.

On many wilderness trips, equipment and supplies are limited by space and weight. This limitation also applies to first aid kits. Wilderness medicine training teaches a care provider to utilize whatever supplies or materials are available, as it is impossible to have optimal equipment to manage all possible situations. Non-medical equipment, such as duct tape and tree limbs, must often be used to fashion splints, and for other medical utilitarian purposes. It is important for first responder students to become familiar with multi-purposing and improvisation, so that they can learn to equip themselves with medical equipment and medications that have the broadest and most practical applications.

Being outdoors is exhilarating. Wilderness sports and activities are refreshing and exciting. The Basic Wilderness Life Support® program is committed to reducing injuries and illnesses in the backcountry. In those situations when misfortune does arise, we seek to hasten the appropriate responses and to increase mitigation through practical, skills-based education and hands-on learning. BWLS® is intended to teach how to become an effective first responder, in order to contribute to the health and well being of all who require medical assistance in the great outdoors.

CHAPTER 1
Patient Assessment

In this chapter you will learn to safely and effectively approach and assess patients in wilderness settings by meeting these objectives:

- Recognize possible threats to rescuer(s) and patient(s) and identify resources through adequately surveying the scene.
- Rapidly determine the presence of any immediately life-threatening conditions while making appropriate interventions during the primary survey.
- Obtain a thorough history and perform an appropriate physical exam as part of the secondary survey.
- Describe the unique component of the Ongoing Survey in a wilderness environment.
- Understand the importance of the following acronyms in pre-hospital patient care: ABCDE, CARTS, AVPU, SAMPLE, OPQRST and C-SPINE.

OVERVIEW

- You are being trained to be a first responder in a wilderness emergency situation. These situations are usually very confusing and very emotionally charged.
- It will be your responsibility to take charge and know how to handle them. The purpose of this chapter is to help you with a process that will allow you to overcome obstacles and provide the patient(s) with the appropriate care.
- This is called first responder medicine.
- Within the professional medical community there are some variations on how to handle a first response but there are important elements to each that will help guide you.
- The process begins by resisting your desire to rush into the situation and assessing the scene.
- Then you will learn the primary and secondary survey, how to develop a problem list, a treatment plan, and finally how to conduct an ongoing assessment.
- The following chart will help explain the process that you will use to assess an injured patient.

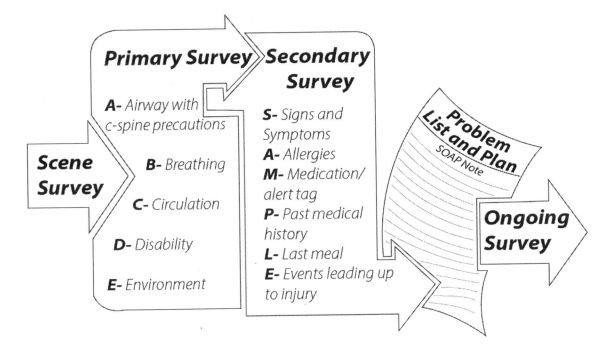

SCENE SURVEY

- The process all starts with surveying the scene.
- The scene survey consists of several parts, the most important of which is safety. Placing a rescuer at undue risk can severely complicate the situation, if not create additional patients. We do not want to create a second victim.
- Surveying the scene also requires the first responder to identify the number of patients; have an understanding of each patient's condition; and note the presence of bystanders, equipment, and other clues that may be useful in determining the **Mechanism of Injury (MOI)** and/or the **Nature of Illness (NOI)**.
- This phase of the patient assessment may also require triage of several patients to effectively utilize limited resources.

Scene Safety

Is the scene safe for me to enter? Consider external hazards such as the following:
- ☐ Physical dangers (rocks, snow/ice, trees, fires, wildlife, etc.)
- ☐ Weather/environment (hot/cold temperatures, lightning, high altitude, etc.)
- ☐ Other people (bikers on single track, climbers above you, hunters, etc.)

Will the scene remain safe? If not, what is my plan?
- ☐ Safe zones
- ☐ Moving patients (drags, carries, and litters)

Is it safe for me to physically care for the patient(s)? **Body Substance Isolation (BSI)** should be considered in *every* patient to prevent disease transmission through bleeding, vomiting, etc.

How many patients are there? Which one(s) need help first? (See Triage section below.)
- ☐ The victim's equipment may provide information about medical conditions or the MOI.
- ☐ Bystanders may have witnessed the victim's demise or may be able to assist with patient care.

Are there resources near the scene that may be useful in treating or evacuating the patient?

Approaching, Identifying, and Getting Permission to Treat the Victim(s)

When approaching the victim, use caution so that you do not expose them to additional hazards such as rock or icefall. Consider marking the route to the scene if additional rescuers are to follow.

Immediately identify yourself as a medical professional and request the victim's permission to treat. If the victim is unconscious or has an altered level of responsiveness, their consent to treatment is implied. Otherwise, the victim has the right to decline treatment.

Ask the victim's name and say "can you tell me what happened?" In addition to defining the MOI/NOI, this will almost always elicit the chief complaint. If the patient cannot answer these questions, they are either unconscious or have an altered level of responsiveness; commence with the primary survey.

This is also an opportunity to determine the Level of Responsiveness (LOR) of your patient. For this we use the **AVPU** (Alert, Verbal Painful, Unresponsive) Scale. Is the patient **A**lert and oriented, responsive only to **V**erbal stimulation, responsive only to **P**ainful stimulation, or **U**nresponsive? If the victim shows any signs of life such as movement, moaning, or talking, then you move on to the primary survey (below). For those victims who are completely unresponsive, the rescuer must quickly move forward into assessment of the ABCs and possibly cardiopulmonary resuscitation (CPR). This is extremely important if the situation involves a lightning strike, submersion injury, or avalanche event with snow burial. These are wilderness situations where immediate CPR may save a victim's life.

Primary Survey: Disability
Level of Responsiveness

A   Alert
V   Verbal – Awakens briefly, withdraws, or moans when spoken to
P   Pain – Awakens briefly, withdraws, or moans in response to painful stimuli
U   Unresponsive – No response to any stimuli

Triage

- When multiple victims are present, it may be necessary to determine the severity of each patient in order to effectively utilize resources.
- Initially, this is done as part of the scene survey by quickly looking over the patients and determining which "look" the worst.
- There are several methods of triaging patients. A common method is to triage them into different color categories based on the victims' severity of illness or injury.
  - ☐ BLACK: Dead on arrival. Patient lacking ABCs despite opening airway.
  - ☐ RED: Critical, immediately life-threatening injury, notable finding during Primary Survey.
  - ☐ YELLOW: Severe injury(s) that is not immediately life threatening.
  - ☐ GREEN: Minor injuries, non-emergent, "walking wounded."
- The color assigned to each patient determines the priority (in order): RED-YELLOW-GREEN-BLACK.
- One key exception is for lightning victims; the BLACK coded patients should be cared for first (see lightning chapter 9).

INITIAL ASSESSMENT

The patient assessment is broken down into 4 parts:

- – Primary Survey
- – Secondary Survey
- – Ongoing Survey
- – Documentation

The urgency to which these parts of the patient assessment decreases from Primary Survey to Documentation however the length of time spent on each section will increase respectively. Additionally, for wilderness based medicine, the importance of complete documentation is really only necessary for very complex patients, patients who's severity is changing with time and in order to follow specific institutional guidelines. You should always consult with your employer or related organization to determine if you have documentation protocols.

PRIMARY SURVEY

Primary Survey: ABCDE

The objective of the Primary Survey is to identify and treat conditions that pose an immediate threat to life. Approaching the victim using the acronym **A B C D E** allows the rescuer to address the life-threatening issues in order of importance. Because this portion of the assessment is searching for critical conditions, it is most applicable to patients who have an altered level of consciousness or have a significant injury. However, this survey should be utilized in *every* victim whom one treats in the wilderness. In those victims who are alert and appear well, this assessment may be brief. Problems found on the primary survey that are life threatening should be addressed immediately, before continuing the survey. It's imperative to remember that even though a patient may have a severe disability from a traumatic event, addressing this comes secondary to ensuring the patient has an **Airway**, is **Breathing** and has intact **Circulation** before addressing their **Disability**.

Primary Survey

A- Airway
B- Breathing
C- Circulation
D- Disability
E- Environment

A– Airway

- There are two issues in the assessment of the victim's airway:
  - ☐ Is the airway currently open?
  - ☐ Is the victim able to maintain their airway?
- First, is the airway open and is the patient able to move air in and out of the airway with minimal obstruction?
  - ☐ If the awake victim is moving air but has sonorous or noisy breathing, then they will generally place themselves in the best position that allows them to keep their airways open. Do not force them into a position that they do not want to go to. Generally, in medicine we like to place victims on their back, but you should not force a victim to this position if they cannot tolerate it.
  - ☐ If the victim has a decreased level of consciousness, then roll them onto their back as a single unit, being careful not to twist or jerk the spine or neck. Once the victim is on their back, then attempt to open the airway using the **head tilt-chin lift** maneuver (illustration below) unless trauma is the MOI.
  - ☐ If you suspect that the victim has head or spinal injuries, use the **jaw-thrust** technique to minimize neck movement by placing one hand on each side of the victim's head and grasping the angles of the victim's lower jaw and lifting up and forward with both hands (photo below).
  - ☐ If the victim with a decreased level of consciousness is not moving air well with initial positioning, then inspect for and remove any foreign objects from their mouth. In victims of avalanches, snow burial, or major trauma, it is not unusual to see snow, teeth, dirt, and leaves in their mouths.
- The second issue is whether the patient is going to maintain their airway throughout the rescue.
  - ☐ There are potential airway issues, especially trauma and allergic reactions, where the patient will have a worsening obstruction to their airway. This is a major consideration when you evaluate evacuation options and the urgency of evacuation for the victims.

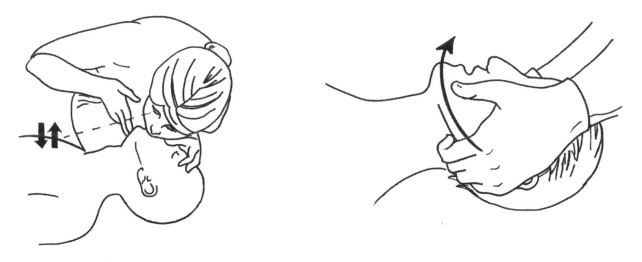

Figure 1.1 Head tilt chin lift   *Figure 1.2 Jaw thrust*

B – Breathing

This involves the evaluation of how well the patient is currently breathing and whether there is any potential respiratory compromise in the future.

- If the victim does not start breathing after the airway has been opened, begin rescue breathing as described for basic CPR using C-A-B as the guide.
  - Each breath should be delivered over one second with enough air to see the chest rise.
  - If the breath does not go in, reposition the airway and try again.
- If the victim is breathing, briefly assess the quality of the respirations. Does the patient appear to be working hard to breathe, is their breathing painful, are they breathing rapidly/slowly, is their breathing appropriate, etc.?

C – Circulation

All patients who are awake or showing any sign of life will have a heartbeat. This step is to assess the victim's cardiovascular status with a focus on the heart rate, pulse strength, and to treat non-massive hemorrhage.

- You can assess the pulse at the radial, brachial, femoral, or carotid arteries.
  - Assess the quality of the pulse. Is it weak/thready, bounding, rapid, or irregular?
  - A general rule of thumb for assessing blood pressure is by the most distal pulse you can palpate. Regardless of the <u>rate</u> of the pulse, if a pulse is present in the following arteries, you can assume that their blood pressure is at least:
    - Pedal pulse = systolic BP of >90mmHg
    - Radial pulse = systolic BP of >80mmHg
    - Femoral pulse = systolic BP of >70mmHg
    - Carotid pulse = systolic BP of >60mmHg
- It's not enough for a patient just to have a pulse. It's also important to ensure that they are not experiencing major Hemorrhage. You can do this by performing a **blood sweep**. This is a rapid (5 - 10 seconds) full, head-to-toe check for blood, wet clothing, swelling, or other signs of bleeding.

A blood sweep affords the rescuer the opportunity to simultaneously note major deformities as well as to evaluate for less obvious sources of bleeding including the 5 potential places where a patient can loose enough blood to be fatal. These locations are remembered by the acronym "**CARTS**" (following page).

D – Disability

Disability serves to remind you to check for neurological status. Is the patient alert, partially alert, or comatose? Is there evidence of cervical spine injury? Treat ALL unconscious trauma patients as if they have a spinal injury until proven otherwise, usually later in the assessment. If the patient is conscious, this is an appropriate time to ask for the mechanism of injury (MOI) to help decide if spinal precautions are necessary. Further harm to the spinal cord can cause serious, permanent disability and death. Also, are there any other major deformities or disabilities?

E – Environment, Exposure and Evacuation decision

At this point in the primary survey, the rescuer has treated any immediate threats to the patient's life and has taken steps to mitigate those threats. Wilderness medicine presents an additional issue that one must consider: the environment and its potential to worsen the victim's medical course.

- Recognize that whatever the environment, the victim has likely been exposed to it for a longer period and has not been compensating as well as the rescuers.
- A victim in a cold/hot environment will be colder/hotter than the rescuer.
- Steps should be taken to limit the victim's exposure to the environment.
- Hypothermia in trauma can lead to increased mortality.
- You must do everything to ensure that the victim remains as warm as possible.
- You should also take this opportunity to Expose the patient by looking under clothes or helmets for additional injuries. Remember that contrary to Urban care, the patient will need their clothes to limit exposure, so NEVER cut or destroy a patients clothing unless absolutely necessary.
- At the end of your primary survey is also the time to determine if this patient necessitates an immediate evacuation, "Load and Go", or if it's suitable to "stay and play."

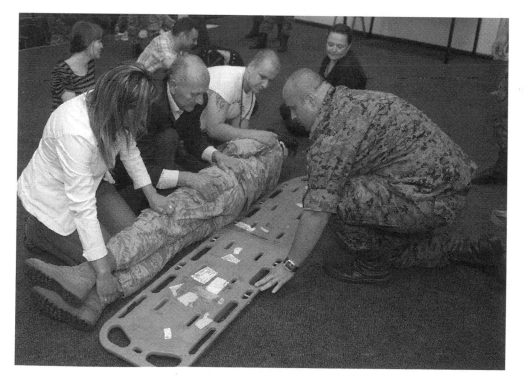

Figure 1.3 Log roll
Photo by U.S. Air Force in Europe

Potential Sources of Major Bleeding

CHEST	The chest is a common source of bleeding, particularly in high-energy trauma. Look for shortness of breath, pain with breathing, and coughing up blood. Examine for chest tenderness, crepitance over the ribs and sternum, flail chest and crackling noises of the chest consistent with air under the skin.
ABDOMEN/PELVIS	Assume abdominal and/or pelvis bleeding in every trauma victim until proven otherwise. Look for bruising over the abdomen and pelvis. Palpate for abdominal and pelvic tenderness on compression.
RENAL	Usually the bleeding is from the kidneys. Look for blood in the urine if you have a prolonged time with the victim. Examine for tenderness of the spine and chest and the lowest level of the ribs.
THIGH	This may occur if there is a femur fracture. Look for deformity, swelling and bruising of the thigh. Palpate for tenderness and crepitance of the thigh.
SKIN/STREET	This is the most obvious place for a rescuer to detect blood. A common error in the wilderness setting is the failure to remove clothing or to roll the patient to look for bleeding. Also, ensure that you survey the area immediately surrounding the victim for a large amount of blood on the ground that may have come from the victim. Specifically an arterial injury that bleeds significantly may be in spasm at the time you are evaluating the victim and not be an obvious source of bleeding.

An exception to the rules of ABCDE

The first objective is to open the airway, however, if a patient is bleeding extensively from a wound, you must first stop this massive hemorrhage rapidly as a victim can lose most of their blood volume in a matter of minutes with major arterial or venous bleeding. In the wilderness, you cannot replace this blood and the victim may be required to be much more active than the typical hospitalized patient.

This step is applicable for only major bleeding and does not include injuries with only minor oozing that will be addressed later in the secondary survey. Generally, these types of injuries are rare in the wilderness but can have fatal consequences if not treated rapidly.

This treatment usually consists of the placement of a tourniquet if it is an extremity injury. If one does not have a tourniquet or if the injury is not amenable to the use of a tourniquet (e.g. facial or torso wound), then a pressure dressing directly on the area of bleeding is the best option.

The placement of the tourniquet does not mandate that the tourniquet stay in place until the patient reaches definitive medical care. The expectation is that that the rescuer will reassess the wound and the bleeding after the patient has been stabilized in the secondary survey and ongoing assessment stage.

Primary Survey in Conscious Patients

■ When the patient is conscious, the rescuer may be able to substitute portions of the complete primary survey with questions. For example:

☐ A talking patient has, for the time being, intact airway, breathing, and circulation. The rescuer should still assess the quality of the breathing and pulse.

☐ Asking a patient about what happened and if they are bleeding may eliminate the need for a blood sweep and spinal immobilization.

CPR – Cardiopulmonary Resuscitation

CPR Guideline Update

The latest American Heart Association guidelines emphasize chest compressions during CPR by re-ordering the initial A-B-C to C-A-B and stating compressions should occur within the first 10 seconds of patient contact.

■ The professional rescuer is still instructed to check for a pulse prior to beginning compressions, while the lay rescuer is advised to only briefly (5-10 seconds) check for signs of movement or breathing.

The compression rate remains 100 per minute with a 30:2 compression-to-breath ratio for adult one- and two-rescuer as well as child/infant single-rescuer.

Two-rescuer CPR for children/infants should be done at a 15:2 compression-to-breath ratio.

The lay rescuer may also elect to employ "hands-only CPR" wherein no rescue breaths are delivered. Note that this should only be done for witnessed adult arrests in urban locations.

Hand positioning remains in the center of the patient's sternum, with a greater emphasis on ensuring adequate compression depth of at least two inches in adult patients and at least one-third of the depth of the patient's chest in children/infants.

Wilderness CPR Considerations

Even in urban settings, CPR with delayed use of an automated external defibrillator (AED), or delayed access to advanced medical care, has success rates that are only 1-6%.

CPR should not be initiated in patients who have obvious signs of death such as lividity, rigor mortis, or decapitation.

Consider that CPR is exhausting to a rescuer, particularly in extreme conditions where energy may be required for self-evacuation. Safety of the rescuers should be considered in decisions regarding duration of CPR attempts in the backcountry.

Current American Heart Association guidelines advise discontinuing CPR in patients who have sustained non-traumatic or blunt traumatic cardiac arrest with the exception of special situations such as lightning or hypothermia after a trial of advanced cardiac life support (ACLS) has been given.

If a patient has been pulseless for longer than 15 minutes, with or without CPR, further attempts at resuscitation should not be made (exceptions are lightning or hypothermia victims).

CPR in the wilderness has the highest success in patients who have been struck by lightning.

A hypothermic patient is "not dead until warm and dead."

These considerations should not prevent initiating CPR in situations where a helicopter or ACLS is accessible within 15-30 minutes, even if a prolonged evacuation may follow resuscitation.

SECONDARY SURVEY

The goal of the secondary survey is to identify and treat any remaining less-critical injuries and illnesses. These conditions may become problems if left unnoticed or if they require advanced medical attention. This portion of the patient assessment is comprised of two key elements:

☐ An abbreviated medical history
☐ A physical exam including vital signs

The individual scenario should dictate the order in which these components are performed. For example, a fallen rock climber should typically have the physical exam portion of the secondary survey performed first to identify any other traumatic injuries, whereas an abbreviated history from a camper who has developed abdominal pain may be more useful. To reinforce the flexibility of the order, we will discuss the physical exam first.

Physical Exam

The physical exam during the secondary survey is a more detailed head-to-toe examination where the rescuer should visibly inspect and palpate the victim from head to toe, including the back.

Vital signs helpful to the wilderness first responder include:

☐ Pulse: in beats/minute, a normal pulse is ~60-100bpm, a high pulse can signify pain or low blood volume
☐ Respirations: in breaths per minute, normal is 12-16 per minute. Rapid breathing can signify a chest injury, or low oxygen, slow breathing can signify brain injury in the proper setting
☐ Blood Pressure (estimated from pulse as mentioned above). A systolic pressure of ~50mmHg is necessary to get blood to the brain and ~70mmHg is necessary to get blood to other vital organs.
☐ Skin color, temperature and moisture (SCTM) can be used to signify heat or cold injuries along with allergic reactions and shock

A general guide for areas to inspect include the following:

☐ Pupils should be equal, round, and reactive to light (**PERRL**).
☐ Blood or fluid draining from the ears or nose suggests a head injury.
☐ Look inside the mouth for loose teeth or other debris that may compromise the airway.
☐ Palpate the cervical spine for tenderness and deformities.
☐ Palpate the chest examining for tenderness, crepitance, and subcutaneous air.
☐ Palpate all four quadrants of the abdomen.
☐ Apply pressure to the pelvis from the top and from the sides.
☐ Examine all four extremities for deformities, tenderness, pulses, and, if the victim is conscious, strength and sensation.

When an abnormality is found, ask the patient if this is an old or new problem, if possible.

Use caution when assessing an area that is suspected to have an injury. Causing pain may impede your ability to obtain an accurate remainder of the exam. You should examine obvious areas of injury last in order to better facilitate your full evaluation of the patient.

When examining an area the patient identifies as painful, begin by assessing above and below the injury, thereby determining the extent of the injury prior to touching the focus of the pain.

Be aware of "distracting injuries" that cause so much pain that the patient does not notice that they have additional injuries. Determining a detailed MOI can help you anticipate other injuries.

Examine the back of the patient at opportune times (e.g. when log-rolling the patient) to minimize movement.

Remember that with an alert and oriented patient, portions of the exam may be substituted for a reliable recollection of the MOI, such as, "I rolled my ankle, didn't fall, and just sat down here on this rock." Such a patient may only require a focused physical exam instead of a complete head-to-toe exam.

Abbreviated History

Most of the patient's history is obtained immediately by asking "what happened?" However, a few other key questions must be answered to ensure proper care is delivered.

The acronym **SAMPLE** will help you to remember the essential points of a patient history.

For critical patients, you may be the only person who gets to talk to the patient while they are conscious, and thus may be the only person who can obtain the history.

Therefore, if an initially unconscious patient regains consciousness, immediately obtain a history.

In patients with an altered level of responsiveness, other clues may be needed to obtain the history. The mnemonic AEIOUTIPS (below) can be helpful in unresponsive patients. A few examples of clues:

☐ Medical alert tags can be found in the form of necklaces, bracelets, anklets, tattoos, etc.

☐ List of medications or medical problems may be found in a wallet.

☐ Medications or devices such as a glucometer (blood sugar meter) or epinephrine auto-injector may be found in a victim's bag/tent/pocket/etc.

☐ Bystanders or family members may be familiar with a victim's past or present medical history.

☐ Cell phones may be employed to contact family members.

To assist you in characterizing a victim's pain, employ the acronym **OPQRST**. Notice that this is most helpful in patients with pain from medical problems rather than traumatic injuries.

Secondary Survey:
A Brief History

S   Signs and Symptoms (chief complaint)
A   Allergies – to anything
M   Medications/ Medical alert tags
P   Past medical / surgical history (illness and injuries)
L   Last meal
E   Events leading up to and causing the accident / injury (what happened?)

Formulating the Assessment:
Altered Mental Status Patients

A   Allergies (anaphylaxis) / Altitude
E   Environment (hyper or hypothermia) / Epilepsy (seizure) – active or postictal
I   Infection (sepsis, meningitis)
O   Overdose (alcohol, medicine)
U   Underdose (medicines)
T   Trauma
I   Insulin (diabetes)
P   Psychological disorder
S   Stroke

Secondary Survey:
Characterizing the Pain

O   Onset: When did the pain start?
P   Provokes/Palliates: What makes the pain better or worse?
Q   Quality: What does the pain feel like?
R   Radiation: Does the pain move anywhere?
S   Severity: How bad is the pain on a scale of 1 – 10?
T   Time: How long has the pain been going on? When did it start?

PROBLEM LIST AND PLAN - SOAP NOTE

SOAP NOTE

SUBJECTIVE
18 year old male, "My ankle hurts"

OBJECTIVE
LOR: alert and oriented x4
HR: 68 and regular
RR: 16
SCTM: pink, warm and dry
BP: radial pulse felt
Pulse: 88
Temperature: not thermometer
Symptoms: right ankle pain
Allergies: allergic to penicillin
Medications:
Past medical history: appendix removed
Last meal: He had 3 hours ago
Events: He slipped, fell 10 feet landing on right ankle, no helmet,
denies loss of consciousness, pain is a 3/10

ASSESSMENT
He has a right ankle injury and possible neck injury

PLAN
Improvised right ankle splint, improvised c-collar, contact SAR
for help evacuating

It is essential that at this point you formulate your thoughts as to what the patient's problems are and how you are going to treat them. There may be many problems or there may be only one. Making a problem list and creating a plan is accomplished using s SOAP note. This is a systematic note that can assist you in creating an assessment and a treatment plan in a backcountry medical emergency.

Subjective: This is information about the patient – often in the patient's own words. "I have been out in the wind for three hours and I am feeling really cold." You can also include Items like age, name, and male or female, adult or child.

Objective: This is information that you gain with your own observations. This is where you will put the SAMPLE history.

Assessment: This is the section where you begin to make a list of what is wrong with the patient.

Plan: For each problem you will write what you are going to do about it.

Once you have created the SOAP note you carry out your plan. However, it should be noted that If the patient is in critical condition, much of this planning is done in your head rather then writing it down. For example, if someone is not breathing you would not waste time to write a SOAP note, rather begin CPR prior to creating a SOAP note.

ONGOING SURVEY

A unique aspect of wilderness medicine is that the rescuer may continue to care for a victim for several hours to days. This wide range of time requires adaptation of the usual patient assessment to include ongoing care. The ongoing survey is heavily dictated by patient's condition, and as such, is quite dynamic.

- Initial vitals obtained during the secondary survey should be compared to vitals taken throughout the evacuation or management period. Changes in vitals help alert the rescuer to an improving or deteriorating patient.
- As changes occur, for example, patient condition, level of responsiveness, or environment, go back to the beginning of the patient assessment.
- If the rescuer has the time and appropriate materials, he or she should try to document the pertinent portions of the evaluation so that this can be handed off to the next level of care so they have a better understanding of the victim's history.

CERVICAL (C-SPINE) ASSESSMENT

When evaluating any patient with known or suspected trauma, there are a number of steps that have to be taken immediately. In addition to scene safety, assessing for major bleeding and airway management already mentioned, you must protect the cervical spine (C-spine). This is performed by grasping the patient's head on each side and holding it steady to make sure the patient doesn't move the neck. This is called "holding C-spine." If the C-spine is injured, any motion of the neck caused by the first responder or the patient may cause serious and permanent injury to the spinal cord. Once you begin holding C-spine, it is imperative that you do not let go until one of three things occurs: 1) you transfer the patient to a higher level of care, 2) you place the patient on a backboard with head restraints or 3) you determine the likelihood of a C-spine injury is very low. The final option is called "clearing" a C-spine. Ideally a doctor in the hospital does this after transport, however, if holding C-spine will significantly complicate an evacuation and professional evacuation is not an option, it's important to know the steps of clearing a C-spine.

The cervical spine may be cleared and immobilization removed from the patient, if the following clinical preconditions are met. First the patient must be fully alert and orientated. The patient must not have used alcohol or drugs that could impair their ability to communicate or reason. There must be no pain over the midline of the back of the neck. There must be no neurological issues, such as numbness or weakness in an arm of leg or any part of the body and no incontinence. Finally, there must be no distracting injury that may 'distract' the patient from complaining about a possible neck pain. A pneumonic that will help the first responder to remember these criteria is "C-SPINE".

- C - cervical midline tenderness
- S - sensory-motor deficit (numbness/weakness)
- P - pain or psychological distractor
- I - intoxication
- N - neurologic deficit (loss of alertness)
- E - events (sufficient mechanism to cause neck injury)

What constitutes 'sufficient mechanism' is not well defined, but someone who falls from a cliff is more likely to have a neck injury then someone who is walking and then twists his or her ankle.

Provided these conditions are met, the neck may then be examined. If there is no bruising or deformity, no tenderness and a pain free range of active motion, the cervical spine can be cleared. The diagnosis of an unstable C-spine injury and its subsequent management can be difficult, and a missed spine injury can have devastating long-term consequences. So be cautious in this analysis. Finally, while it is tempting to focus on the cervical spine, it is important to assess and clear the entire spinal column as well. It is also important to remember that commercial C-collars or those improvised from SAM splints or clothing are only to serve as a reminder to the patient not to move their neck, they do not actually provide complete cervical stabilization.

QUESTIONS

1. **What is the purpose of the blood sweep during the primary survey?**
   a) To clear the scene of blood by sweeping it away with a broom
   b) To identify sites of major bleeding
   c) To detect major deformities
   d) All of the above
   e) B and C only

2. **You are rock climbing with several of your friends when there is a rock slide and three of your friends fall 10 to 20 feet to the bottom of the cliff. There are also two other people who were injured by falling debris soon afterwards while standing at the bottom of the cliff and looking up. Which one of the following is correct in terms of managing this situation?**
   a) You should move all of the injured people away from the base of the cliff.
   b) You should not move anybody as there is a risk of spinal injury by moving them.
   c) You should put an overhead shade over those at the base of the cliff but not move them.
   d) You should triage the injured, only moving those without concern of spinal injury from the base of the cliff.
   e) You should leave all patients where they are lying and leave immediately to get help.

3. **A hiker falls down a steep embankment 150 feet and lands at the bottom. She is pale but awake. She has a thready carotid pulse of 130 beats / minute and complains of feeling very thirsty. Which one of the following best explains her increased heart rate, paleness, and thready pulse?**
   a) Abrasions on her lower legs and hands that are dirty but have no active bleeding
   b) Deformity of her left wrist without any significant swelling
   c) Deformity, pain, and swelling in her right ankle
   d) Neck pain and stiffness
   e) Severe tenderness on palpation of her abdomen

4. **Which one of the following is NOT correct in regards to obtaining a history from a patient in the secondary survey?**
   a) S = Signs and Symptoms
   b) A = Allergies
   c) M = Medications
   d) P = Past medical history
   e) L = Last meal
   f) E = Exposure to elements

5. **You are three days into a weeklong backpacking trip when one of your group develops worsening abdominal pain. After performing a thorough assessment (including history), you suspect constipation to be the cause and elect to watch the patient overnight. How frequently should you reassess the victim?**
   a) Every 5 minutes all night
   b) Every 15 minutes
   c) Just reassess in the morning
   d) Never, you already made your assessment
   e) Whenever a change in patient condition or environment occurs

6. **Which one of the following is NOT an area that is concerning for occult blood loss in the trauma victim?**
   a) Abdomen
   b) Buttocks
   c) Chest
   d) Pelvis
   e) Thigh

7. **You are snowshoeing in the mountains during winter. It has been in the mid 20s most of the day. You come upon a 35-year-old man off to the side of the trail. He is breathing and has a strong regular pulse but is very confused and slow to respond to you. He does not complain of anything. Which one of the following is a potential etiology for his altered mental status?**
   a) Hypoglycemia due to too much insulin
   b) Seizure with a post-seizure confusion
   c) Stroke
   d) Intoxication with alcohol
   e) All of the above should be considered

8. **You arrive at the scene of a submersion (drowning) event. The victim has been pulled from the water and is lying on his back. On your initial assessment the victim is completely unresponsive without any sign of life. Which one of the following is the most appropriate next step in the management of the victim?**
   a) Evaluate for massive hemorrhage and place a tourniquet if necessary.
   b) Initiate CPR with chest compressions.
   c) Initiate CPR starting with two-rescue breaths.
   d) Perform a blood sweep.
   e) Start rewarming the patient using blankets and body heat.

9. **Which one of the following is not correct for the Primary Assessment?**
    a) A – Airway
    b) B – Breathing
    c) C – Circulation
    d) D –Drugs
    e) E – Environment

ANSWERS

1. e 2. a 3. e 4. f 5. e 6. b 7. e 8. c 9. d

CHAPTER 2

Airway and Breathing

Objectives:

- Understand the importance of an open airway and how it can become obstructed in trauma situations.
- Learn how to open and maintain an airway in adults and children.
- Learn how to remove a foreign object obstructing a patient's airway.
- Review rescue breathing techniques in adults and children.

Case

While you are sitting around a campfire enjoying a freshly roasted marshmallow, two people come frantically running into your campsite. They say that when they were climbing up a rocky ledge 20 yards away from your campsite, a rock came loose and struck their friend. You quickly run to the scene and begin your primary assessment. You immediately notice the girl is not breathing.

- What should you do in this case?
- What are some ways you can open her airway?
- What other precautions should you take while trying to open this girl's airway?

After clearing the scene for environmental hazards, prepare to approach the patient and open her airway.

1. Gently tap the patient and ask if she is okay.
   - ☐ Avoid shaking the victim since her spine has not been cleared of injury.
2. Place the patient in the supine position.
   - ☐ Do this by rolling the person while stabilizing the neck and putting it in continuous traction.

If there is an object in the patient's mouth, a finger sweep can be used to remove it. Note that a finger sweep should not be used with infants.

The patient's heart will stop within a few minutes if the patient is not breathing. If the heart is not induced to beat within four to six minutes, irreversible brain damage will occur. That is why every wilderness first responder MUST know how to clear and maintain an open airway. Quick treatment is crucial!

THE AIRWAY

An open airway signifies that air is able to flow freely from the nose or mouth to the bronchioles in the lungs. The tongue often blocks the airway in cases where the patient is unconscious and in the supine position.

One of three maneuvers can be used to open the airway:
1. Head-Tilt/Chin-Lift Maneuver
2. Tongue-Jaw Lift Maneuver
3. Jaw-Thrust Maneuver

Head-Tilt/Chin-Lift Maneuver

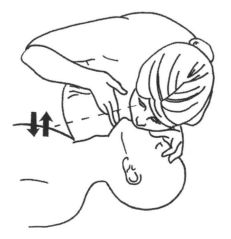

Figure 2.1 Head-Tilt/Chin Maneuver

1. Tilt the head back by placing pressure on the forehead and lift the chin as shown.
2. When lifting the chin, apply upward pressure on the bone (avoid pressing on the soft tissue below as this may further block the airway).
3. Continue until chin points to sky. In children, place head in neutral position.

Tongue-Jaw Lift Maneuver

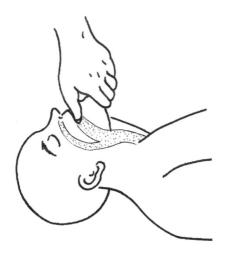

Figure 2. 2 Tongue-Jaw Lift Maneuver

The tongue-jaw lift maneuver is used to remove an object that is lodged in the mouth.
1. Grasp the tongue and lower jaw between your thumb and finger.
2. Lift the jaw up and out.

Jaw-Thrust Maneuver

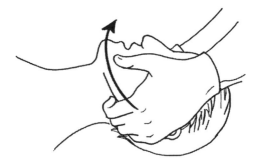

Figure 2.3 Jaw-Thrust Maneuver

1. Kneel at the victim's head facing the victim's feet.
2. Put arms in such a position that creates a continuous line with the patient's spine.
3. Place thumbs on cheekbones and two or three fingers at the corner of the patient's jaw (at the angle between chin and ear).
4. Use counter pressure from your thumbs on the patient's cheekbones.

☐ Assess the patient's breathing.
☐ Look, listen, and feel for air movement with your ear and cheek.
  ☐ Look for the rise and fall of the patient's chest.
  ☐ Listen and feel for breath from the patient's mouth.
☐ A breathless patient requires foreign-body removal and/or rescue breathing.
☐ Please note that when doing the jaw thrust maneuver the neck and spine are put in traction. Once in traction, the neck must remain in traction, which can be achieved by applying a SAM splint or by continually holding the neck. That means that it is preferable to have two people when doing the jaw-thrust maneuver so as to further assess the patient.

Foreign-Body Airway Obstruction: Conscious Adult (Heimlich Maneuver)

1. Wrap arms around the person's waist from behind (keep elbows out from ribs).
2. Make a fist and place thumb in on midline abdomen above navel and well below the bottom of the sternum (xiphoid process).
3. Grab your fist with your second hand and pull quickly in and up in a powerful motion.
4. Repeat until airway clears or until the patient goes unconscious.

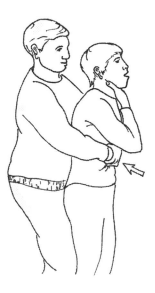

Figure 2.4 Heimlich Maneuver.

Foreign-Body Airway Obstruction: Conscious Adult Lying Down

1. This technique is called the abdominal thrust.
2. If the patient is not in the supine position, roll them onto their back paying extra attention to the neck.
3. Kneel astride the patient's thighs.
4. Place the heel of your hand on the patient's midline abdomen above the navel and below the sternum.
5. With your second hand on top of your first, press in and upward with a powerful motion.
6. Repeat thrusts until airway clears or patient goes unconscious.
   ☐ For pregnant women, follow protocol for abdominal thrust except perform thrusts against the patient's chest with your hands on the *middle* of the sternum.

☐ For children ages one to eight, open airway with tongue-jaw lifts and remove object **if seen**.

☐ **DO NOT** perform blind finger sweeps or the object may be lodged deeper in the airway.

Foreign-Body Airway Obstruction: Unconscious Adult Supine Position

1. Open airway with the tongue-jaw lift maneuver. Do a finger sweep along the cheek, the base of the tongue, and the opposite cheek.
2. Perform the head-tilt/chin-lift maneuver and ventilate by sealing your mouth over the patient's mouth, pinching the patient's nostrils and breathing out so the patient's chest rises. If this fails, reposition airway and try a second time.
3. If the airway is still blocked, straddle the patient's thighs and give five abdominal thrusts.
4. Repeat steps 1-3 until the patient's airway is opened.
5. Once the airway is open, and if the patient still has no breath, start rescue breathing.

Foreign-Body Airway Obstruction: Conscious Infant Less than One Year Old

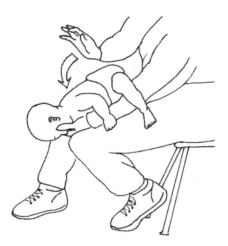

Figure 2.5 Foreign-Body Airway Obstrution in Conscious Infant less than 1 Year Old

1. Determine why there is a lack of breath (look, listen, and feel as described above).
2. Hold infant as shown in the image above, supporting the head with the head positioned lower than the trunk.
3. Give five forceful blows between shoulder blades with the heel of your hand.
4. Using the hand that was used to give the blows, support the neck and back of the baby's head while turning the baby supine, then give five chest thrusts with the finger of your free hand on the lower half of the baby's sternum.
5. Repeat until the breathing is clear or until the baby is unconscious.

Foreign-Body Airway Obstruction: Unconscious Infant Less than One Year Old

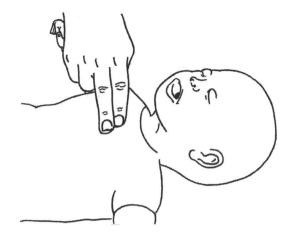

Figure 2.6. Foreign-Body Airway Obstrution in Unconscious Infant less than 1 year old

1. Open the airway using tongue-jaw lift maneuver. Look for obstruction—**DO NOT** blind finger sweep.
2. Open the airway and ventilate by sealing your mouth over the patient's mouth **and nose** and breathe out so the baby's chest rises.
3. If the first attempt fails, reposition the airway and try a second time.
4. If the airway is still blocked, give five back blows then five chest thrusts.
5. Repeat steps 1-3 until the airway is opened.
6. If the baby is still not breathing once the airway is open, start rescue breathing.

Heimlich Exceptions Review

- Standing adult—come from behind.
- Supine adult—perform abdominal thrusts.
- Unconscious patient—give finger sweep and two attempted rescue breaths before abdominal thrusts.
- **DO NOT do a blind finger sweep in children.**
- Use tongue-jaw thrusts to open airway in children and look for obstruction.
- Infants receive back blows first and then abdomen thrusts.

Rescue Breathing Review

1. Pinch the patient's nostrils and hold the mouth open.
2. Take a deep breath away from the patient's mouth.
3. Seal your mouth over the patient's mouth.
4. Give two full, **SLOW**, forceful breaths making sure to see the chest rise.
   - ☐ Too much air too quickly forces air into the patient's stomach, which is not good because the victim may vomit.
5. If you cannot see the chest rising, reposition the airway and try again.
   - ☐ Note that a second failure means the airway is blocked.

6. Check for pulse. If it is present, continue breathing.
    ☐ If there is no pulse, start CPR.
7. Use one breath per five seconds.
8. Rescue breathing can be done mouth to mouth or mouth to nose if necessary.

Rescue Breathing Exceptions in Children and Infants

1. Do not fully extend the victim's head to open the airway.
    ☐ Full extension blocks the airway.
2. Seal off mouth and nose with your mouth.
3. Use small puffs instead of full breaths.
4. Watch the patient's chest and abdomen.
5. Use one breath per three seconds.
    ☐ Too much air too quickly will cause gastric distention and may impede filling of lungs.
    ☐ Only remove air from stomach by pressure if absolutely necessary.
    ☐ Patient may vomit and clearance of vomit in recovery position will be necessary.
    ☐ To put the patient in the recovery position roll the patient "as a unit" while supporting the head. Point patient's nose "downhill."
    ☐ If you must, leave the patient propped into position (with backpacks, logs, etc.).

QUESTIONS

1. **When preparing to open an airway, what is the first thing you should do?**
   a. Tap on the person and ask if they are okay. Move the person into the supine position.
   b. Move the person onto his or her side and press their chin into their chest.
   c. Give the person a good shake to see if you can get them to gain consciousness.
   d. Move the person to a sitting position, then rotate their head from side to side to see if any objects protrude from their throat.

2. **A person has a foreign body obstructing their airway and you decide to perform the Heimlich maneuver. Which of the following is not a step?**
   a. Place the heel of your hand on the patient's midline abdomen above the navel and below the sternum.
   b. With your second hand, grasp throat and check for position of foreign object.
   c. With your second hand on your first hand, press in and upward with powerful motion.
   d. Repeat thrusts until airway clears or the patient goes unconscious.

3. **Which of the following maneuvers do you use to open the airway of a person whom you suspect has a spine injury?**
   a. Head-Tilt/Chin-Lift Maneuver
   b. Tongue-Jaw Lift Maneuver
   c. Jaw-Thrust Maneuver

4. **In a conscious infant who is six months old, which of the following is NOT a step in the process of removing a foreign body from the airway?**
   a. Determine lack of breath.
   b. Hold infant with trunk lower than head.
   c. Give five forceful blows between shoulder blades with heel of hand.
   d. Make baby sandwich with other arm, turn baby supine, and give five chest thrusts with finger of your free hand on the lower half of the baby's sternum.

ANSWERS
1. a 2. b 3. c 4. b

CHAPTER 3
Bleeding and Shock

Objectives:

- Understand the dangers of bleeding and demonstrate how to control bleeding using various techniques.
- Be able to describe specific causes, stages, and symptoms of shock.
- Be able to demonstrate how to manage a patient in shock.

Case

You are mountain biking outside Yosemite National Park when one of your friends falls violently on a rocky downhill section of trail. As he stands back up to dust himself off, you notice lots of blood running from his right thigh. He has landed on a sharp rock in the trail that has cut deeply into his inner thigh. Bright red blood is pouring from the laceration.

■ What would you do?
■ An understanding of bleeding and how to control life-threatening bleeding is one of the most **critical** intervention techniques the first responder must learn.

All bleeding stops – eventually – but you want to make sure it stops before the patient dies.

Life depends on a continuous flow of blood.

The average adult has four to six liters of blood.

The Heart

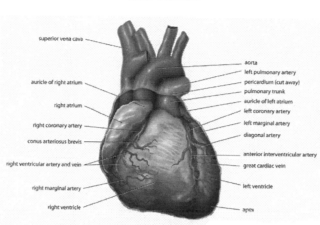

Figure 3.1. The Human Heart

The heart is a huge muscle that acts as a pump to supply blood to the rest of the body. It is very oxygen dependent.

Tracking Blood Flow

☐ (From large to small): heart – arteries – capillaries – veins (and then back to the heart)

HEMORRHAGE: BLEEDING FROM A WOUND

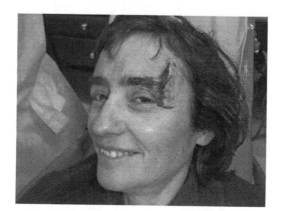

Figure 3.2 Head Wound

Hemorrhages are not exclusive and can be internal or external. Hemorrhages are classified by the type of vessel that has been injured. The following list helps to identify what type of vessel has been injured:

Capillary bleeding – slow oozing and bright red

- Venous bleeding – steady flow and dark maroon (due to low oxygen in veins)
- Arterial bleeding – under high pressure, often spurting and brighter red

Vasoconstriction is the body's automatic response to bleeding. Within seconds of an injury, vessels constrict and small blood cells called platelets stick to the torn wall of the vessel. This congregation of platelets initiates a cascade of events by which clotting factors cause bleeding to slow or stop.

Most capillary and small venous hemorrhaging will stop bleeding without your assistance. However, larger wounds and arterial damage will usually require outside control to stop the bleeding.

Control of External Bleeding

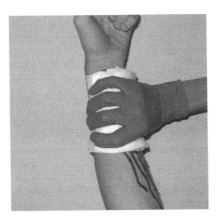

Figure 3.3 – Pressure to Control External Bleeding

- The most immediate concern that you need to consider is how quickly blood is being lost. In most cases of external bleeding, the first method of control is to apply direct pressure on the wound.

  1. When applying direct pressure, remember to follow these rules:
     - ☐ Use gloves and sterile dressing (if available) to reduce the chance of infection.
     - ☐ Apply pressure with the heel of hand directly onto wound for 10-20 minutes.
     - ☐ Be patient.

- Certain wounds are particularly hard to control. Large wounds, because of the extensive vasculature involved, and scalp wounds, because of tension pulling in opposite directions leaving the vasculature open, are especially difficult to control.

  2. The next step is to elevate the wound.
     - ☐ Assure this is done as soon as possible.
     - ☐ Raise the wound above the level of the heart as this reduces blood pressure to the injured extremity.

  3. A pressure bandage may also be used if:
     - ☐ There is persistent bleeding
     - ☐ You need to free up your hands in order to treat the wound more effectively.
       - When applying a pressure bandage, use bulky dressing and elastic wrap.
       - After applying a pressure bandage, be sure to check distal function and pulse often.

4. Pressure points can also be used to control bleeding.
   - ☐ These are points of the human body under which major arteries pass.
   - ☐ There are two main pressure points: Brachial and femoral pressure points.
   - ☐ Be sure to press the artery against bone to slow blood flow.

Using a Tourniquet

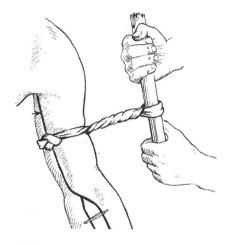

Figure 3.4 Using a Tourniquet

While widely viewed as a last resort, a tourniquet can be used initially for a short interval of time to determine the best approach of treatment and evacuation. If you decide to use a tourniquet in this fashion, do not leave it for more than a minute or two.

If you have tried the other methods to stop the bleeding this is now being used as a last resort.

Apply tightly and proximal to wound.

Always note the time the tourniquet was applied. (Writing the time on the victim's forehead is very effective.)

Avoid loosening once in place.

If you use a tourniquet, you have determined to sacrifice the limb in order to save the life.

INTERNAL BLEEDING

Bleeding into a body cavity is life-threatening.

■ Patients can bleed to death internally in specific areas of the body (CARTS):
   - ☐ Chest
   - ☐ Abdomen
   - ☐ Renal/Retroperitoneal
   - ☐ Thigh
   - ☐ Street

Patient may go into shock before you are aware of any bleeding.
   - ☐ Carefully assess injuries to CARTS and any unexplained signs of shock.
   - ☐ Look for external bruising, guarding, and an increasingly rigid abdomen.

There is little treatment that can be done while in the field for internal bleeding.
- ☐ Stabilize injuries.
- ☐ Treat for shock.
- ☐ Initiate rapid evacuation.

SHOCK

Shock is defined as the lack of blood flow to vital organs, especially the brain.
If blood flow is not maintained to the brain, shock, coma, and death can result. The heart, blood, and blood vessels are responsible for maintaining blood flow to the brain.

Causes of Shock

All shock results from failure of one or more of the components of the cardiovascular system.
Cardiogenic Shock
- ☐ Failure of the heart
- ☐ Heart attack – muscle damage due to lack of blood supply
- ☐ Trauma to heart

Hypovolemic Shock
- ☐ Caused by a low fluid volume, occurs with severe bleeding, dehydration, and burns.
- ☐ With severe bleeding, remember CARTS.

Vasogenic Shock
- ☐ Caused by low resistance to blood flow within blood vessels. This means that the vessels enlarge causing the blood pressure to decrease, and the heart cannot maintain blood flow.
- ☐ Occurs with spinal injuries, infection (septic shock), and allergies.

Symptoms of Shock

Each stage is usually indicative of the amount of blood that has been lost.
Stage 1: Compensatory Shock
- ☐ Anxiety, confusion, restlessness, pale and cool skin
- ☐ Increased pulse and respirations
- ☐ Normal or even elevated blood pressure
- ☐ Patients showing these declines in vital signs should be <u>evacuated</u>.

Stage 2: Decompensatory Shock
- ☐ Altered level of consciousness, cold and clammy skin
- ☐ Rapid weak pulse and respirations
- ☐ Decreased blood pressure (hard to find a pulse)
- ☐ At this point, the patient may be saved with RAPID EVACUATION.

Stage 3: Irreversible Shock
- ☐ Drowsy, unresponsive, cold skin
- ☐ Slow heart rate and slow, labored respirations
- ☐ No pulses palpable
- ☐ At this point, most patients will die or suffer damage to vital organs even with evacuation.

Special Risk Factors of Shock

- ■ Children and young adolescents
  - ☐ In the case of children and young adolescents it can be hard to tell that they are in shock as their bodies tend to be more resilient and compensate for a longer period of time against signs of shock, essentially masking the severity of the condition.

- ■ Elderly
  - ☐ Elderly are the opposite of children and young adolescents, as their bodies do not compensate as well and have an even earlier onset of shock.

- ■ Diabetics
  - ☐ Diabetics have an increased risk of dehydration.

- ■ Pregnant Women
  - ☐ The fetus is endangered due to diverting of blood to abdomen during shock.

Management of Shock

Anticipate and treat for shock until you have ruled it out.

1. Early intervention will slow the downward spiral.
2. <u>Avoid panic</u> – *your calm attention may be all that keeps your patient alive.*
3. Any anxiety can worsen shock (Psychogenic Shock)
4. Treat the underlying cause (when possible).
5. Stop bleeding, splint fractures.
6. Elevate legs above head (no more than 10 to 12 inches).
7. Insulate from cold or protect from heat.
8. Monitor vital signs every five minutes.
9. Orally rehydrate.
10. Transport ASAP.

Evacuation Guidelines

Initiate *immediate, rapid* evacuation for all patients suspected of going into shock.

Review

1. Direct pressure, elevation, and pressure points help to stop or slow bleeding.
2. Remember to check for internal bleeding (CARTS).
3. Shock occurs when there is a lack of blood to vital organs (especially to the brain).

4. Determine why the patient is in shock.
5. Symptoms
   - ☐ Confusion
   - ☐ We were given pulses so we could check for shock!
6. Management
   - ☐ Keep people hydrated
   - ☐ Be looking for it
   - ☐ Be calm
   - ☐ Treat causes
   - ☐ Elevate legs
   - ☐ Maintain body temperature
   - ☐ Monitor vitals
   - ☐ Orally rehydrate
   - ☐ Evacuate

QUESTIONS

1. **Which of the following describes blood flowing from a venous hemorrhage?**
   a) slow oozing and bright red
   b) high pressure, often spurting and brighter red
   c) steady flow and dark maroon
   d) bubbling and very thin

2. **Which of the following is NOT a method of treating shock?**
   a) Insulate from cold or protect from heat
   b) Avoid giving liquids so as to not overload the body
   c) Elevate legs above level of head
   d) Transport immediately

3. **How many liters of blood does the average adult have in their body?**
   a) 4-6L
   b) 7-9L
   c) 10-12L
   d) 2-4L

4. **Which of the following describes Stage 1 of compensatory shock?**
   a) Altered level of consciousness with cold/clammy skin and decreased blood pressure and decreased pulse
   b) Anxiety, confusion, restlessness, and pale/cool skin with increased pulse and respirations
   c) Drowsy, unresponsive, and cold skin. Slow heart rate and slow labored respirations
   d) Heightened alertness, unequal pulses, dilated pupils, and heavy respirations

5. **Which of the following is NOT a body area/cavity usually associated with being able to bleed to death into?**
   a) Renal/retroperitoneal
   b) Thigh
   c) Chest
   d) Throat

ANSWERS
1. c 2. b 3. a 4. b 5. d

CHAPTER 4

Vitals Workshop

Objectives:

- Review the steps of a primary assessment.
- Learn the significance of vital signs and what they measure.
- Practice obtaining vital signs from a conscious and unconscious patient.

Case

On a rock-climbing trip, you and a friend who is a physician come across a man who has fallen from a steep precipice. You check to verify that the scene is safe and immediately assist the physician in the primary assessment.

Primary Assessment

Airway- The patient is breathing shallowly and the airway seems to be open. Your friend instructs you to keep the airway open using the jaw-thrust technique and to stabilize the patients cervical spine.
Breathing- The patient is taking slow shallow breaths

Circulation- Your friend detects a radial pulse. The patient is bleeding form a large laceration on the top of his head. There is no other bleeding.

Disability- The patient is unconscious and unresponsive.

Environment- It is eighty degrees Fahrenheit and you are one mile from the trailhead.

The physician begins a secondary survey by checking the patient's heart rate, respiration rate, and his pupils. What do these vital signs tell him?

Vital Signs

What are vital signs?

The word "vital" refers to items that are essential for life in a body.

Vital signs are the measurements of these items.

They are essential to measure early in the assessment of a patient and include the following:

1. Level of consciousness (LOC)
2. Heart rate (HR)
3. Respiration rate (RR)
4. Skin color, temperature, and moisture (SCTM)
5. Blood pressure (BP)
6. Pupils (P)
7. Body core temperature (T)

When should you take vital signs?

Take (and record) a patient's vital signs as part of the physical exam. Continuously monitor patients until they are no longer under your care.

Consecutive sets of vital signs will tell you how the patient is doing.

Have the same rescuer take the vital signs to prevent variability.

In the wilderness, the second set of vitals is often more important than the first, the third set is more important than the second, etc.

Make sure you document the exact time each set of vital signs was taken.

Early-changing vital signs

Level of consciousness

Heart rate

Respiration rate

Skin color, temperature and moisture

☐ These vital signs will change QUICKLY if a patient is in trouble.

Late-changing vital signs

Blood pressure

Pupils

Body core temperature

☐ Changes in these vital signs may indicate a more serious condition.

Level of Consciousness

- Measure of the brain's ability to relate to the outside world
- Often the FIRST vital sign to noticeably change
- Can be the most difficult to assess accurately

Measurement of LOC

- A - Alert
- V - Verbal
- P - Pain
- U - Unresponsive

Alert

- The patient is alert and able to answer questions appropriately.
  - ☐ What's your name?
  - ☐ Where are you?
  - ☐ What day is it?
  - ☐ What happened?

Verbal

- The patient is not alert but does respond in some way when spoken to.
  - ☐ Grimacing
  - ☐ Grunting
  - ☐ Rolling away from rescuer
- The patient may be able to follow simple commands.

Pain

- The patient does not react to verbal cues but does react appropriately to painful stimuli.
- Appropriate responses to pain:
  - ☐ Pulling away from rescuer or pushing rescuer away
  - ☐ Groaning or moaning
- Inappropriate response to pain:
  - ☐ Curling into a fetal position is indicative of a deeper level of unconsciousness

Unresponsive

- Patient does not respond to stimuli.

Heart Rate

The heart rate can be taken anywhere you can palpate a pulse (a pressure wave created by the beating of the heart).

The radial pulse is usually the easiest to check.

Heart function can be assessed in a patient by checking the heart rate, the heart rhythm, and the quality of each heartbeat.

Rate = number of beats per minute
- ☐ Normal = 60-100 bpm in adults. Children typically have a higher heart rate with newborns ranging from 100-150 bpm.
- ☐ Count pulse for 15 seconds and then multiply by four.

Rhythm
- ☐ Regular
- ☐ Irregular

Quality = Force the heart exerts with each beat
- ☐ Normal
- ☐ Thready – weak, indicates inadequate circulation
- ☐ Bounding – abnormally forceful

Respiratory Rate

Rate = number of breaths/minute
- ☐ Breathing in AND out counts as one breath.
- ☐ Normal = 12-20 bpm
- ☐ Count for 15 seconds and multiply by four.
- ☐ Measure the respiratory rate WITHOUT the patient knowing. An easy way to accomplish this is to pretend like you are taking the patient's pulse while secretly counting the respirations.

Rhythm
- ☐ Regular
- ☐ Irregular

Quality
- ☐ Normal = quiet/effortless/easy/unlabored
- ☐ Abnormal = suggests that something may be wrong
  - Too shallow or unusually deep
  - Pained
  - Wheezing, gurgles, gasps
  - Nostril flaring

Skin Color, Temperature, Moisture

Color

Look at the color of the patient's skin in non-pigmented areas (lining of eyes, inside of mouth, and fingernail beds). Pink skin is the normal color in these non-pigmented areas.
- Red or flushed skin
  - ☐ Vasodilation (widening of blood vessels)
  - ☐ May indicate fever or hyperthermia
- White or pale skin
  - ☐ Vasoconstriction (narrowing of blood vessels)
  - ☐ May indicate shock or hypothermia

Blue skin or cyanosis
- ☐ Indicates a lack of oxygen in blood

Yellow skin or jaundice
- ☐ May indicate liver failure

Temperature

Check skin temperature with the back of your hand.
Check skin INSIDE of clothing, not on exposed face or hands.

Moisture

Normal skin is slightly moist but feels relatively dry.
Cool and moist skin may indicate shock.
Hot and dry skin may indicate hyperthermia.

Blood Pressure

Blood Pressure = the pressure exerted by the blood against the walls of the blood vessels, especially the arteries, as it circulates through the body
- ☐ Normal 90-150/60-90 mm Hg

Ways to measure blood pressure:
- ☐ Sphygmomanometer (cuff) and stethoscope
- ☐ Sphygmomanometer alone
- ☐ Blood pressure by estimation

Sphygmomanometer and stethoscope.
Wrap the cuff snugly around the patient's arm one inch above the elbow.
Line up indicator with brachial artery. This can be identified towards the inside of the patient's arm in the elbow region.
Palpate the brachial pulse.
Make sure the patient is sitting upright, legs uncrossed, with the cuff positioned at the level of the heart.
Inflate cuff until you can no longer feel the radial pulse.
Inflate the cuff another 20 mm Hg.
Place the stethoscope diaphragm over the brachial artery.
Deflate the cuff 2-4 mg Hg per second.

Systolic blood pressure

The needle reading when you HEAR the first heart sound
Is the force exerted against the arterial walls by the blood when the left ventricle contracts

Diastolic blood pressure

The needle reading when you hear the last heart sound
The blood's pressure against the artery when the heart is at rest

Sphygmomanometer alone

  Palpate the radial pulse.

  Inflate the cuff while still palpating the radial pulse.

  Deflate the cuff slowly, noting on the dial of the cuff the point at which the radial pulse returns.

  This is the patient's systolic blood pressure.

  Note that this technique is only applicable for measuring systolic blood pressure. Diastolic blood pressure cannot be measured without a stethoscope.

Estimating Blood Pressure:

If pulse is present, systolic blood pressure is greater than the following:

  Carotid Pulse – 50 mmHg

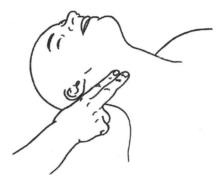

Figure 4.1.Feeling a carotid pulse

  Femoral Pulse –60 mmHg

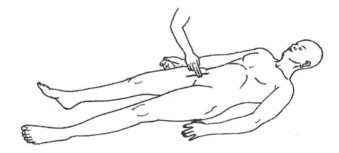

Figure 4.2. Feeling a femoral pulse

  Brachial Pulse - 70 mmHg
  Radial Pulse – 80 mmHg

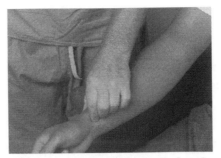

Figure 4.3 Feeling a radial pulse

Pedal Pulse – 90 mmHg

Pupils

Pupils should be equal, round, and reactive to light (PERRL).
- ☐ Constrict with exposed to light
- ☐ Dilate when light is reduced

Unequal pupils or those that do not respond to light may indicate a head injury.

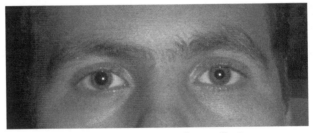

Figure 4.4 Unequal pupil size

Both pupils should constrict and dilate equally.

Body Core Temperature

Thermometers that are not always accurate in wilderness:
- ☐ Glass thermometers can be damaged by extreme heat or cold.
- ☐ Standard thermometers do not register hypothermia-range temperatures.
- ☐ Axial (armpit) temperatures are notoriously unreliable.

Normal – 98.6 degrees F (37 degrees C)

Oral temperature
- ☐ Easy access and accurate
- ☐ Minimal discomfort

Rectal temperature (make sure to use a rectal thermometer)
- ☐ Most accurate in children or infants who are unable to hold a thermometer safely in their mouths
- ☐ More difficult to access
- ☐ More discomfort

Recording Vital Signs:

- [ ] LOC = AVPU
- [ ] HR = 50-100 bpm, regular, strong
- [ ] RR = 12-20 breaths per minute, regular, unlabored
- [ ] SCTM = pink, warm, dry
- [ ] BP = 90-150/60-90 mm HG
- [ ] Pupils = equal, round and reactive to light (PERRL)
- [ ] Temp = 98.6 degrees F

QUESTIONS

1. **Which of the following changes in vital signs is most consistent with a serious, life-threatening condition?**
   a) A blood pressure change of 5 mmHg
   b) A pupil on one side that is larger than the other
   c) A respiration rate that changes from 16-20 over the course of four hours
   d) Skin that changes color six hours after blunt trauma

2. **Which of the following vital signs will change quickly if the patient is in trouble?**
   a) Body temperature
   b) Level of consciousness
   c) Heart rate
   d) All of the above

3. **When measuring the level of consciousness of a patient and they seem to respond to you when you ask them to roll over and can grunt and groan but not much else, where would they fall on the grading scale?**
   a) Alert
   b) Verbal
   c) Pain
   d) Unresponsive

4. **If you are able to measure the femoral pulse of an unconscious patient but are unable to feel their brachial pulse, what is the most likely range for their systolic blood pressure?**
   a) At least 50mmHg, but less than 60mmHg
   b) At least 60mmHg, but less than 70mmHg
   c) At least 70mmHg, but less than 80mmHg
   d) At least 80mmHg, but less than 90mmHg

ANSWERS
1. b 2. d 3. b 4. b

CHAPTER 5

Abdominal and Chest Injuries

Objectives:

- Describe the basic anatomy of the abdomen and chest.
- Describe the general signs and symptoms of abdominal and chest injuries.
- Describe the general treatment for abdominal and chest injuries.
- Demonstrate specific treatment for blunt and penetrating abdominal trauma.
- Demonstrate specific treatment for chest trauma.

ABDOMINAL TRAUMA

Case 1

You are camping in the mountains when you hear a friend scream. When you get to her, you notice that she has fallen off of a large rock, landing on a small boulder. She is complaining of abdominal pain and holding her abdomen.

The abdomen is commonly separated into four quadrants that are used to help diagnose the origin of the abdominal pain and locate internal organs.

Right upper quadrant (RUQ)
Right lower quadrant (RLQ)

Left upper quadrant (LUQ)
Left lower quadrant (LLQ)

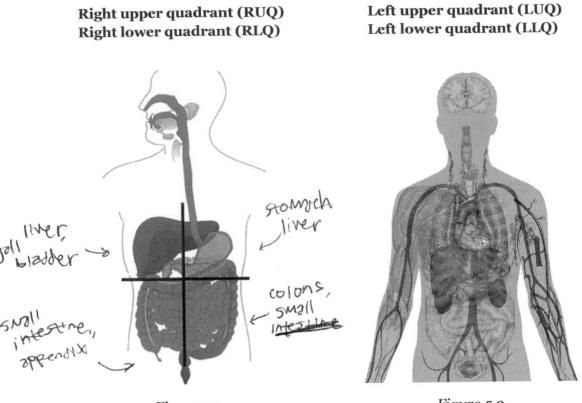

Figure 5.1

Figure 5.2

The RUQ contains:

Liver, right kidney (lies closer to the back than the abdomen), gall bladder, and duodenum
Also contains part of the pancreas and transverse colon

The LUQ contains:

Liver, stomach, left kidney (lies closer to the back than the abdomen), pancreas, transverse colon, and spleen

The RLQ contains:

Small intestine, ascending colon, appendix, right ureter, and bladder (possible)
In females the right lower quadrant also contains the following:
Right ovary, Fallopian tube, Uterus

The LLQ contains:

Small intestine, descending colon, sigmoid colon, left ureter, and bladder
In females the left lower quadrant also contains:
☐ Left ovary, left fallopian tube, uterus (if enlarged), abdominal organs

Hollow versus Solid Organs

The abdominal organs are usually divided into solid or hollow organs. The solid organs are the pancreas, liver, spleen and kidney. All other organs, such as the intestines and bladder are hollow organs. This knowledge has ramifications on how injuries are treated.

Steps of an Abdominal Assessment

- Determine the mechanism of injury (MOI).
- Upon knowing the mechanism of injury, determine what kind of damage could have been done.
- Does the mechanism of injury indicate possible injury to the abdomen or merit concern?
- Is the patient moving or staying still?
- Does the patient appear to be in a great deal of pain?
- Look at the patient's abdomen while they are lying down.
- Look for symmetry as well normal shaping of the abdomen.
- Look for signs of trauma such as the following:
- Penetrating wounds
- ■ Bruising
- Feel the abdomen by gently applying pressure in each of the four quadrants.
- Look for signs of pain, tenderness, firmness, rigid muscles, and lumps.
- Listen to the four abdominal quadrants with a stethoscope or your ear. Bowel sounds (gurgling) should be present.
- Monitor vitals signs. If there is internal bleeding, the patient could go into shock.
- Ask the patient if they have had blood in their urine, stool, or vomit as this can indicate internal bleeding.

Trauma

There are two types of trauma that need to be ruled out in an abdominal assessment:
1. Blunt trauma
2. Penetrating trauma

Blunt trauma

Usually occurs from a forceful blow to the abdomen. First determine the mechanism of injury and events leading up to the injury. Ask the patient and/ or bystanders to give you a description of the accident as this can give you an idea of what injury the patient could have sustained. Always assume the worst-case scenario before clearing an injury. Be sure to remember your anatomy, such as distinguishing solid organs like the liver or spleen and hollow organs like the small intestine.

Performing a general abdominal assessment:
- ☐ Be especially aware of bruising.
- ☐ When feeling the abdomen, feel for unusual lumps.
- ☐ Be aware of the abdomen swelling and also becoming more firm (due to internal bleeding).
- ☐ See if the patient "guards" against pressure in any quadrant during the assessment.
- ☐ Be caring during the assessment.

☐ Look for problems with solid organs, such as internal bleeding that can lead to shock.
☐ Be aware of peritonitis.
☐ Check for rupture of the abdomen or internal organs.

*Peritonitis is an inflammatory reaction within the abdomen. It is described as a sharp, stabbing, or burning pain. The patient will be in a considerable amount of pain, so much that they will not want to move. In order to alleviate the pain by decreasing pressure on the abdomen, the patient may assume the fetal position.

Signs and symptoms of abdominal injuries
☐ Nausea and vomiting
☐ Blood in the patient's urine, stool or vomit
☐ Increased respirations and elevated heart rate
☐ Fever may develop, especially if patient develops peritonitis
☐ Reddened skin at the site of the injury

Treatment of abdominal injuries
☐ Follow the ABCDE guidelines
☐ Keep patient still and warm
☐ Avoid giving the patient anything to eat or drink
☐ If it is a long evacuation, patient may have small sips of a cool liquid
☐ Do not give the patient alcohol

Penetrating Trauma

Occurs when an object passes through or penetrates into the abdomen.
Severity depends mainly upon what organ(s) is injured (remember your anatomy).
1. Bleeding can be lethal. If your patient is in shock or going into shock, their only chance of survival depends on immediate evacuation.
2. If patient is stable and doesn't need immediate evacuation, infection is now a bigger concern.

Assessment: Same as for a blunt trauma.
Treatment:
☐ Generally the same supportive care as you do for blunt trauma
☐ Specific treatment depends on the degree of soft tissue injury
☐ Control bleeding
☐ Clean all wounds
☐ Do not remove impaled object

Evisceration: This is when the intestines protrude out of the injured site.
☐ Remove all clothing from around the wound
☐ Apply a bandage soaked in clean as water over the exposed intestine.
☐ Apply another layer of dressing to prevent the dressing from drying out.
☐ Cover with a thick dry dressing.
☐ Check every two hours to be sure the inner dressing is moist
☐ Evacuate immediately.
☐ If evacuation is going to be long, intestines may be gently pushed back into the abdomen after being cleaned with a sterile wash.

CHEST TRAUMA

Case 2

A young man falls while hanging food in a tree – he falls, scraping his arms and legs. He quickly develops shallow breathing because it hurts on the side of his chest. You notice blood in that same area and pull back the shirt to see a superficial cut. There is point tenderness. He is alert. The bleeding is superficial, and while he has painful breathing it is not getting worse. His chest expands equally on both sides.

Anatomy of the Chest

- Twelve ribs on each side protect the chest. It needs this protection because so many vital organs are found in this area.
- All the ribs are connected to the thoracic spine in the back, the top 10 ribs are connected in the front to the sternum either directly or by cartilage, while the bottom two 'float' in the chest wall.
- The lungs fill both sides of the chest, also called the thoracic cavity. The right lung has three lobes the left lung has only two because the heart pushes into that side of the chest.
- On the bottom of the thoracic cavity is a domed muscle that appears like a shelf – called the diaphragm. This is the main muscle that causes humans to breathe. There are other muscles that are in between the ribs, called the intercostal muscles that expand the rib cage and help, usually with heavy breathing.
- When a person takes in a breath, the diaphragm drops down, expanding the chest cavity, causing a decrease in pressure. Air rushes to fill this void. This is called the active phase of breathing. When the diaphragm relaxes, air is pushed back out through in what is called the passive phase of breathing.

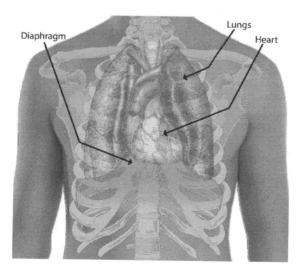

Figure 5.3 Anatomy of the Chest

Common Chest Injuries

Chest injuries are common. Most are not serious, but some are life threatening. When you examine someone for a chest injury there are several important points to remember.

- Examine the chest - Look for blood, bruising, or broken skin.
- Look at the rate and depth of breathing – is the patient breathing faster or more shallow?
- Look at the ease of breathing - is the patient having more trouble breathing?
- Look at the sputum (saliva) – is there blood in the saliva?

A patient that has point tenderness on the chest wall and is breathing much faster and is also having trouble breathing should make you aware of a more serious situation requiring fast action. It the patient is also coughing up blood this would heighten your concern even more.

Fractured or injured rib

- The most common chest injury
- Usually not life threatening
- A fractured rib can puncture a lung so watch for this
- These are very painful and there is point tenderness over the injury site
- Patients breathing is usually more shallow because of the pain
- Often there will be bruising at the site of injury
- Watch for signs of punctured lung (pneumothorax - mentioned below)
- Treatment is mostly supportive
- Patients with minor fractures need little done
- Wrap chest with a swathe to help manage pain. This is particularly helpful if the patient is coughing or needs to sneeze. You can use a shirt, towel or sheet
- Anti-inflammatory medicines such as ibuprofen will be useful
- Sometimes putting the arm on the affected side in a sling helps – but this is problematic in the back country if the patient needs to use that arm
- If symptoms worsen, consider one of the more serious conditions below

Flail Chest

- This occurs when 2 or more consecutive ribs completely fracture causing this section of the chest to move inward when the patient breathes in and move outward when a patient breaths air out
- This is paradoxical to normal rib motion
- The broken ribs are called a "flail"
- This is usually life threatening
- Bruising is usually seen and blood might also be seen at the injury site
- Watch for this paradoxical motion of the chest wall
- Treatment
  - ☐ This injury requires immediate evacuation
  - ☐ There is little treatment in the field that can be undertaken, but you can try to place a bulky dressing over the flail, tape midline to midline, If symptoms worsen—remove the dressing.
  - ☐ Evacuate with injured side down or as most comfortable.

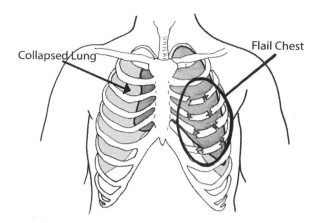

Figure 5.4 Flail Chest

Pneumothorax

Literally this means "air in the chest"

Signs and Symptoms:
- ☐ Sharp chest pain
- ☐ Increasing difficulty breathing
- ☐ Increasing anxiety
- ☐ Rapid pulse
- ☐ Bruising
- ☐ Pale, cool, clammy skin (signs of shock)

Treat similar to rib fracture:
- ☐ Oxygen if available – descent in altitude
- ☐ Semi - reclining is usually a better position
- ☐ Immediate evacuation

Tension Pneumothorax

This is the result of a pneumothorax

Extremely life threatening

Air keeps leaking from lung on the side of the pneumothorax

Lung is compressed to about the size of a tennis ball

Heart is then compressed and can stop beating

Great vessels leading into the heart are compressed or kinked

This can causes the jugular veins in the neck to distend

Opposite lung can also become compressed.

Trachea may deviate toward uninjured side

Breath sounds may diminish or stop on the side of the injury

Signs and symptoms of a tension pneumothorax are more severe than a regular pneumothorax
- ☐ Distended neck veins
- ☐ Tracheal deviation
- ☐ Falling blood pressure

- ☐ Sharp chest pain
- ☐ Increasing difficulty breathing
- ☐ Decreasing level of consciousness
- ☐ Rapid pulse
- ☐ Pale, cool, clammy skin (signs of shock)
- Treatment
  - ☐ Immediate evacuation

Sucking chest wound

- Penetration of chest
- Hole in chest wall
- Bubbling sound while breathing
- Air moves in and sometimes out of hole
- Air sucked through the hole collapses the lung
- Signs and Symptoms:
  - ☐ Difficulty breathing
  - ☐ Moist sucking sound /bubbling
  - ☐ Increasing anxiety
  - ☐ Rapid Pulse
  - ☐ Pale, cool, clammy skin (shock)

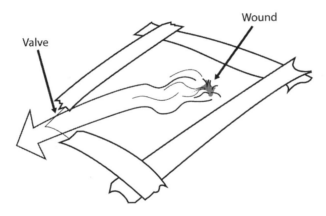

Figure 5.5 Treatment for Sucking Chest Wound

- Treatment:
  - ☐ Plug the hole with a glove or piece of plastic
  - ☐ Leave one corner free so that air can exit but not enter.
  - ☐ If air doesn't leave then a pneumothorax can develop and the patient can stop breathing

Hemothorax

- Broken ribs can tear a vessel and cause blood to collect around the lung in the pleural space
- This can be very serious
- Blood can pool around the lung and prevent expansion of lungs
- Breath sounds may diminish

May see blood in sputum (hemoptysis)

Signs and Symptoms
- [ ] Sharp chest pain
- [ ] Increasing difficulty breathing
- [ ] Increasing anxiety
- [ ] Rapid pulse
- [ ] Possibility of hemoptysis
- [ ] Pale, cool, clammy skin

Treatment - evacuation if it is suspected, there is nothing that can be done in the field

Pericardial Tamponade

Can be caused by blunt or sharp trauma to the chest

Blood and fluid collects around the heart in the pericardial sac, compressing the heart

Difficult for heart to pump blood

Treatment - Evacuation if it is suspected, there is nothing that can be done in the field

General Chest Injury Guidelines

Keep Airway open

Inspect bare chest: look, ask, feel

Treat any injury
- [ ] Stabilize fractures
- [ ] Close open wounds

Supplemental oxygen if you have access to it or decent in altitude if possible

If possible let patient get comfortable

Avoid medicines that suppress breathing

QUESTIONS

1. **Which of the following is found in the right upper quadrant (RUQ)?**
   a) Liver, right kidney, gall bladder, and duodenum
   b) Small intestine, ascending colon, appendix, right ureter, and bladder
   c) Small intestine, descending colon, sigmoid colon, left ureter, and bladder
   d) Stomach, left kidney, pancreas, transverse colon, and spleen

2. **You are biking in Moab when you come across a man who is clutching his abdomen. He said he crashed on his bike half an hour ago and the handle bars were thrust into his abdomen. He has bruising in his right upper quadrant and is in significant pain. What should you do?**
   a) Ask the man to try walking and see if you can give him some food.
   b) Keep the man still and warm as you look for an evacuation route. Avoid food and water.
   c) Use your wilderness medical kit to find the man some pain medication. If none is found, alcohol can be ingested to dull the pain.
   d) Wrap a tight bandage around his abdomen to keep his innards in place.

3. **A person falls landing on his chest. He has immediate pain. Within a few minutes he begins to have extreme shortness of breath, increased chest pain, distended jugular veins in his neck, and a deviated trachea. His most likely diagnosis?**
   a) Cardiac Tamponade
   b) Pneumothorax
   c) Tension pneumothorax
   d) Flail chest

4. **While backpacking, you come across a woman who fell from a tree and landed on a branch below, causing a small branch to penetrate her abdomen in the lower left quadrant. She seems alert and is having only moderate amounts of pain. When you observe the wound, you are not sure how far it has penetrated but it is bleeding a moderate amount. What is the most worrisome immediate complication that should be addressed?**
   a) Gastrointestinal upset
   b) Bleeding
   c) Infection
   d) Pain

ANSWERS
1. a 2. b 3. c 4. b

CHAPTER 6

Altitude Illness

This chapter describes how to recognize, prevent, and treat health conditions caused by high altitude.

Objectives:

- Recognize the signs and symptoms of acute mountain sickness, high altitude cerebral edema, and high altitude pulmonary edema.
- Understand that gradual assent is the key to preventing altitude illnesses.
- Understand that the most important treatment for altitude illness is descent.
- Become familiar with additional methods for both preventing and mitigating altitude illnesses.

Case

A 38-year-old attorney from New York City, USA decides to take a ski trip to Colorado. He flies into Denver and then rents a car and drives directly to his accommodations at a ski resort at about 9000 feet (3000 meters) That night he finds that he sleeps poorly and awakes with a splitting headache. Attributing his headache to his restless night, he takes some acetaminophen, drinks his coffee, and heads to the rental shop to get set up for a day of skiing. On his way to the rental shop, he becomes nauseated and runs to the men's room to vomit. He then decides that he must have eaten something wrong the night before and decides to head to the resort's medical clinic where he meets you.

1. What is your recommendation for the treatment of this patient?
2. Does he need to fly home to New York and abandon his hard-earned trip, or can he stay and wait through his illness?
3. What symptoms would you expect if his condition worsened?

HIGH-ALTITUDE ILLNESS

High-altitude syndromes are usually only seen at altitudes in excess of 2000 meters (6560 ft). Two major issues affect the human body above this altitude. Frist the brain will start to swell. The result is acute mountain sickness (AMS) that will progress to high altitude cerebral edema (HACE) if not treated. The other major affect is that the lung can fill with fluid. The result is called high altitude pulmonary edema (HAPE). These are the three major syndromes of altitude illness and are considered a failure to acclimatize.

Acute Mountain Sickness (AMS)

Minor brain swelling
A thorough history is the key to the diagnosis of AMS as there are no specific physical exam findings.
The key piece of information is the amount of elevation gain and the rate of elevation gain.
AMS is a common illness that may occur in 10-70% of individuals depending primarily on the rate of ascent.
Headache is a necessary symptom in order to diagnose AMS.
In addition to headache, at least one of the following features needs to be present:
☐ Dizziness
☐ Fatigue
☐ Nausea/vomiting
☐ Insomnia
☐ Lack of appetite

Treatment

Discontinue ascent and rest.
Take Acetaminophen and ibuprofen for headache.

Increase oral fluid intake as tolerated.

Administer supplemental oxygen if available.

Descent is definitive treatment.

High Altitude Cerebral Edema (HACE)

As the brain continjes to swell the symtpoms worsen. HACE represents a progression of AMS to the point of life-threatening brain damage. HACE is defined as severe AMS symptoms plus additional symptoms as follows:

Unsteady gait

Altered level of consciousness

Severe lassitude

While the boundary between AMS and HACE can be blurry, and HACE can develop quickly, HACE almost never occurs without antecetent AMS symptoms. The progression of AMS to coma typically occurs over one to three days.

Treatment

IMMEDIATE descent (almost always with assistance) is imperative and should not be delayed unless descent poses a greater danger to the parties involved (i.e. weather, terrain, etc.). Even modest elevation losses can be helpful.

Oxygen supplementation should be given if available.

If descent is not possible, place patient in a portable hyperbaric chamber for four to six hours.

Recovery is likely to be prolonged with some symptoms (unsteady gait) lasting up to weeks. Most who survive eventually fully recover.

High Altitude Pulmonary Edema (HAPE)

Plasma, the liquid component of blood can leak into the lung tissue. This is called high altitute pulmonary edema (HAPE). HAPE usually evolves over two to four days after ascent to altitude. The primary symptoms are the following:

Shortness of breath at rest

Rapid heartbeat

Cough

Exercise intolerance

Possible bluish discoloration around the lips

Possible crackles over lung fields.

Occasional pink frothy sputum that is produced when coughing (usually occurs later in illness)

HAPE may be seen with co-existing HACE. Mild cases may resolve within hours after descent. In contrast, severe cases may progress to death within 24 hours, particularly if descent is delayed.

Treatment

- IMMEDIATE descent is imperative (likely with assistance as exertion will worsen symptoms). Descending 500-1000 meters (1500-3000 ft) may be all that is required before improvement is observed.
- Administer supplemental oxygen.
- Rest after descent.
- If descent is not possible, place the patient in a portable hyperbaric chamber (if available).
- Neither supplemental oxygen, hyperbaric therapy, nor any other intervention should delay an opportunity to descend.

PREVENTION OF HIGH-ALTITUDE ILLNESS

- Graded ascent is the safest method to facilitate acclimatization and prevent altitude sickness.
- The most important factors in developing altitude illness are how high and how fast you ascend, the altitude at which you sleep (sleeping altitude), and your genetic makeup.
- Current recommendations for climbers without experience at high altitude are to spend two to three nights at 2500-3000 meters (8,000-10,000 ft) before further ascent.
- Increases of greater than 600 meters (2,000 ft) in sleeping altitude should be avoided and one should consider an extra night of acclimatization every 300-900 meters (1,000 to 3,000 ft). For example, if you spent the previous night at 15,000 ft, then you may hike higher than 17,000 ft the following day, but must descend below 17,000 ft to sleep.
- Modest evidence suggests that Ginko biloba is effective in preventing acute mountain sickness.
- Medications can be prescribed by physicians familiar with altitude travel that can help prevent AMS, such as acetazolamide, and dexamethasone.

EVACUATION RECOMMENDATIONS

With all altitude-related illness, the definitive treatment is always descent. However, descent is not the same as evacuation. In select circumstances patients with altitude-related illness can descend for a period of time while their bodies acclimatize before re-ascending.

Acute Mountain Sickness:

- Patients with AMS need not necessarily be evacuated. Resting at the current altitude and receiving symptomatic treatment may be sufficient for complete recovery within 24-48 hours.
- Extreme caution should be used if the patient is to continue to ascend as symptoms can progress to HACE.
- Patients should be symptom free for at least 24 hours before attempting to ascend again.

High Altitude Cerebral Edema:

- Patients with HACE should be evacuated after descent.
- Patients with HACE are not safe to attempt re-ascent on the current expedition.

High Altitude Pulmonary Edema:

- Patients with HAPE should be evacuated.
- Death from HAPE can proceed rapidly, and descent followed by evacuation should not be delayed.
- Some climbers with mild HAPE (characterized by dry cough and mild shortness of breath at rest) may be reluctant to abort an expedition as these trips usually represent thousands of dollars of investment. As a medical provider, in extremely mild cases, you can advise them to descend until symptom free and then wait for a period of days for further acclimatization. However, if symptoms return upon re-ascent after a second period of acclimatization, that person should be evacuated.

QUESTIONS

1. **What is the factor that most greatly predisposes people to altitude-related illness?**
   a) Genetic predisposition
   b) Fitness level
   c) Altitude
   d) Rate of ascent
   e) Alcohol intake

2. **Which of the following are considered appropriate treatment options for acute mountain sickness?**
   a) Acetaminophen
   b) Ibuprofen
   c) Rest and discontinuation of ascent
   d) Descent
   e) All of the above

3. **Which of the following is <u>not</u> a feature of high altitude pulmonary edema?**
   a) Rapid heartbeat
   b) Cough
   c) Unsteady gait
   d) Rapid breathing
   e) Bluish discoloration of the lips

4. **High altitude cerebral edema differs from acute mountain sickness in which of the following ways?**
   a) Headache is only seen in AMS.
   b) Vomiting is only seen in HACE.
   c) Unsteady gait is commonly seen in AMS.
   d) Patents with AMS can be confused or stuporous.
   e) Altered mental status and unsteady gait are hallmarks of HACE.

ANSWERS
1. d   2. e   3. c   4. e

CHAPTER 7

Avalanche Survival

This chapter discusses the fundamentals of avalanche safety, rescue, and survival.

Objectives:

- Describe and recognize terrain and snow conditions that predispose to avalanche.
- Understand the utility of avalanche safety and survival tools.
- Recognize that the time to recovery is the most significant factor for victim survival.
- Describe the most appropriate way to organize a rescue.
- Understand the types of injuries caused by avalanche burial.

Case 1

Just prior to the season's opening of a ski resort, you and a group of three friends decide to take advantage of recent snowfall by hiking up the mountain with your skis and snowboards to get some "fresh tracks." While all of you are experienced, you are the only person familiar with the local terrain.

1. What preparations need to be made before departure to improve the safety of your trip?
2. What are the essential tools you need to carry?
3. Describe the type of route you wish to select to safely lead your friends up the mountain.
4. When it is time to descend the mountain, what safety measures will be taken?

Case 2

After getting to the summit and enjoying lunch, you and your three friends are prepared to descend the mountain. One member of your party decides to hike a few hundred feet farther along the ridgeline so that he can ski down the center of the bowl. When he is skiing within the bowl, the snow starts to move with him and then suddenly collapses under him. He is swept down the mountain in the ensuing avalanche. You try to keep sight of your friend as long as possible as he tumbles down the mountain, but as the snow settles and stops, you are only able to identify a ski pole and a mitten on top of the debris.

1. What are some of the greatest threats to your friend's survival?
2. Describe how you and your two remaining friends will organize yourselves to try to rescue the victim.
3. What risks do you need to be mindful of while attempting to rescue the victim?
4. Describe how you would use various avalanche safety and survival tools to improve the victim's chance of survival.

BACKGROUND

Facts

- Injury and death due to avalanches have dramatically increased over the past two decades.
- Asphyxiation is the predominant mechanism of death among avalanche victims.

As many as one-third of avalanche victims sustain significant blunt trauma.

Hypothermia is a rare cause of death among avalanche victims.

■ *The most important factor in avalanche survival is the amount of time buried in the snow.*

Depth of burial is the second most important factor in avalanche survival.

Avalanches can be predicted by snow conditions and terrain.

In the vast majority of avalanche burials, the avalanche was triggered by the victim or someone in the victim's party.

Avalanches can reach speeds of up to 100 mph in less than 10 seconds.

Snowmobilers account for the largest group of back country users who are killed in avalanches.

50% of avalanche victims who are completely buried die within the first 20 minutes of burial.

Noise does not trigger avalanches.

Avalanche Types

1. Slab Avalanches

Most avalanche accidents occur from slab avalanches. Slab avalanches occur when two layers of snow, such as granular snow on smooth snow, do not adhere to one another. This allows the top layers of snow to fracture as a unit. Since the instability is between two layers of snow beneath the surface, the danger is often invisible.

Clues such as sinking, cracking, or collapsing snow should alert you to instability.

2. Wet Snow Avalanches

These avalanches occur anytime there are prolonged periods of elevated temperatures that warm up the snow surface. This is more common in the spring.

They primarily occur in the afternoon, after the sun has had time to melt the top several centimeters of the snow surface.

They are slower moving; however, high density and heavy slides can drag victims over rock formations and cliffs, even if the slide is small.

3. Powder Avalanches

Powder avalanches start as a single point and grow as they progress.

These are the fastest of the three avalanche types. When large and fast enough, avalanches can send shock waves in advance of their descent, increasing the amount of destruction in the path of the avalanche.

Factors That Predispose to Avalanche

1. Weather

Strong winds carry snow and deposit dense unstable layers on lee slopes. These thick deposits can shear and carry massive amounts of snow down in a snow slide.

Extended periods of melting of the snow pack make slabs more likely to avalanche.

Any recent heavy snow falls, particularly when the snow falls on old snow that has gone through freeze/thaw cycles.

2. Terrain

- Exposed slopes with few trees are more prone to avalanche.
- Slope angles greater than 30 degrees, and less than 55 degrees, are more likely to avalanche..

PATHOPHYSIOLOGY

General

The pathophysiology of death by avalanche follows the sequence of *trauma, acute airway obstruction, early asphyxia (lack of oxygen), late asphyxia*, and *hypothermia*.

Trauma

- Up to one-third of avalanche victims have massive trauma as either the primary cause of death or as a major contributor to their death.
- Multiple injuries, such as spinal and long bone fractures, blunt abdominal trauma, and closed head injuries, are sustained as the avalanche victim is dragged over rocks and through trees.
- Primary protection from brain trauma through the use of helmets in the wilderness is recommended.

Acute Airway Obstruction

- Inhalation of snow by the avalanche victim results in rapid asphyxiation if the victim is unable to clear his or her airway as the snow slide slows.
- Acute airway obstruction or acute asphyxiation is responsible for the immediate drop in survival observed after 15 to 30 minutes of burial.
- If an avalanche burial victim is extricated within 15 minutes, chances of survival are greater than 90% but drop to 30% as time to extrication approaches 35 minutes.

Early and Late Asphyxia

- If chest movement is not restricted to the point of compromising breathing mechanics, survival depends on the size of the air space created by the victim's face as the snow flow slows.
- All air pockets will ultimately fail for two reasons:
  - ☐ Heat from the expired air causes an ice lens to form on the air-snow interface, preventing continuous gas exchange.
  - ☐ Rebreathing the same air will eventually use up all the available oxygen and lead to death from asphyxiation.

Hypothermia

- Avalanche victims die from trauma or asphyxiation far sooner than they die from hypothermia.

While hypothermia can significantly increase the morbidity of the victim, it is the primary cause of death in less than 2% of avalanche victims.

The rate of core cooling is unlikely to cause life-threatening hypothermia before 90 minutes of burial.

AVALANCHE SAFETY AND SURVIVAL

Safety

Education is the key to avalanche avoidance. Specific field instruction with avalanche professionals is encouraged. Alternatively, travel with a guide who is knowledgeable in avalanche safety and who can recognize danger.

When traveling, never travel directly above any member of your party.

Avoid "terrain traps," such as gullies and narrow valleys. These serve as run-out zones where avalanches far up the mountain can funnel through, burying everything on the bottom of the gully.

Travel from one safe zone to another one person at a time. If an exposed area needs to be crossed, never expose more than one person at a time. Keep the rest of the party in a safe area so that they can perform a rescue if an avalanche occurs.

Be on the look out for "red flags," such as collapsing or cracking snow or sinking into wet snow.

Start on low angle slopes, which are less than 30°, before venturing to steeper slopes. This will give you the opportunity to better assess snow stability before traveling on the higher risk steeper slopes.

When skiing or snowboarding through avalanche-prone terrain, always go one person at a time.

Use releasable bindings so that if caught in an avalanche your skis don't trap you at the bottom of the debris (the "anchor" effect).

Let someone at home know where you have gone and when they can expect you to return.

Always call the Forest Service or Avalanche Forecast Center for a report of the current snow safety.

Always carry avalanche rescue equipment, including at a minimum an electronic avalanche rescue transceiver (beacon), shovel, and probe and practice using them. Also, consider using other safety equipment that is currently (or soon) available including the AvaLung from Black Diamond Equipment Limited, the Air Ball from K2, and avalanche air bags, which are expected to be introduced in the United States in the near future.

Wear a helmet.

Survival

If caught in an avalanche, attempts should be made to remove all ski equipment including skis and poles.

Backpacks may be left on as they may provide some measure of spine protection.

Attempt to "swim" to the surface of the debris.

As the snow slows, the most important thing to do is get a hand or both hands in front of the face to create and protect an airway and air pocket around the face

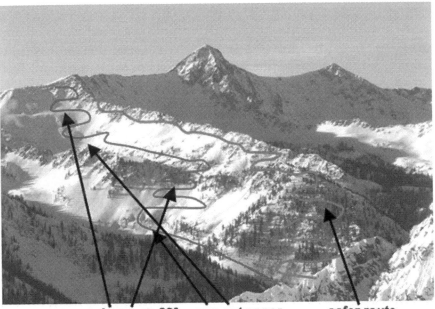

exposed areas > 30°   run out zones   safer route

Figure 7.1 Dangerous vs. Safer Routes to Avoid Avalanche

AVALANCHE VICTIM RESCUE

- If an avalanche is witnessed, the survivors should make every effort to maintain sight of the victim as he/she is pushed down the slope.
- Once the survivors lose sight of the victim, a mental note should be made of the area where the victim was last seen using fixed landmarks such as rocks and trees.
- As more than one avalanche is possible in the same area, extreme caution should be used by the rescuer to avoid getting caught in a second avalanche. One member of the rescue party should be designated as the team leader and should stand at a safe distance away from the debris and other rescuers and look out for potential danger.
- Transceivers (beacons), shovels, and probes constitute the basis of avalanche survival and rescue equipment. Transceivers work on the assumption that an avalanche victim can be found within the "golden 15 minutes" after burial (after 15 minutes, the chances of survival dramatically decrease).
- If a member of a party is buried in an avalanche, rescuers should switch their transceivers from the "send" to the "receive" mode. This will allow rescuers to pick up the signal transmitted by the victim's beacon without interference from the other members of the group.
- Using a systematic pattern, rescuers can hone in on the victim's signal with their receiving transceivers.
  - ☐ A rule of thumb is to start at the place where the victim was last seen and work "downstream," making wider and wider switchbacks as you travel down the avalanche path.
  - ☐ Leave surface clues such as gloves and ski poles in place where you found them so that other rescuers can probe around them or walk around them with a transceiver to see if a signal is picked up in the area around the articles.

- ☐ Once the maximal signal is obtained on the lowest sensitivity setting, then the transceiver is placed on the snow where the signal is strongest and rescuers start to probe in a grid-like fashion around the signal.
- ☐ Once a body is felt with the probe, leave the probe in place and dig the snow out around the probe, using caution as to not further injure the victim with the shovel.
- ☐ If multiple victims are involved, turn off the victim's transceiver once he is extricated so as to not interfere with the signal of another victim's transceiver.

TREATMENT

- Asphyxiation is the major threat to life in avalanche victims.
- ■ As with any victim, primary attention should first be given to the ABCs.
  - ☐ If the victim is not breathing spontaneously, clear all snow and debris that may be obstructing the airway and listen for breathing sounds.
  - ☐ If the victim is still not breathing spontaneously, then initiate rescue breathing. If resistance is met, reassess for airway obstruction.
  - ☐ Continue the primary assessment and treat as discussed in the Patient Assessment chapter.
- Because major trauma frequently accompanies avalanche burial, cervical spine precautions should be used when extricating the victim. Immobilize the victim on an improvised litter made from skis and other material if necessary.
- If lethal injuries are present at the time of extrication, then attempts at resuscitation are not recommended.
- Resuscitative efforts should continue on a victim without a pulse who was buried more than 45 minutes if an obvious air space is identified at extrication.
- Continue with the secondary assessment as previously discussed.
- Keep in mind the patient's exposure to the environment. Snow can be insulating. Once the victim is extracted from the snow and exposed to wind, core body cooling can accelerate if the body is not properly insulated against the environment.

EVACUATION GUIDELINES

- Any avalanche burial victim should be evacuated immediately.
- The entire party should turn around and discontinue the trip if there is any concern at all for potential avalanches.
- If on a multi-day tour or if caught in a storm such that evacuation poses as much risk as proceeding on the trip, then the involved parties should stop and make every reasonable effort to find shelter in a safe area (such as digging a snow cave in a heavily wooded area) until the storm clears and a safe route can be navigated.

QUESTIONS

1. **Which one of the following is the most important determinant of avalanche victim survival?**
    a) The ability of the victim to create an air pocket around his or her face
    b) The fitness level of the buried victim
    c) The length of time for which the victim is buried
    d) The victim's ability to remove skis and poles before burial
    e) Type of avalanche in which the victim is caught

2. **When traveling over snow in the wilderness, which one of the following guidelines should be observed?**
    a) Exposed areas are frequently safest as there is less risk of being injured against a tree.
    b) Gullies and narrow valleys are generally safe places to travel.
    c) Safer slopes are generally between 35 and 45 degrees.
    d) Talk in low, hushed voices so as to not disrupt an avalanche.
    e) Travel one person at a time when crossing hazardous areas.

3. **When performing a rescue for an avalanche victim, which one of the following is true?**
    a) Rescue efforts should stop after 35 minutes because there is little chance for survival after this time.
    b) Rescuers should turn their transceivers from "receive" to "send" mode.
    c) More than one avalanche in the same area is rare.
    d) Cervical spine precautions should be observed when extricating avalanche victims.
    e) Hypothermia is the biggest concern with avalanche victims.

4. **If caught in an avalanche, which of the following should be attempted?**
    a) Create an air pocket around the mouth and face.
    b) "Swim" to the surface.
    c) Ski to the side of the slide.
    d) Remove skis and poles.
    e) All of the above.

5. **You are snowshoeing along a sturdy ridge when directly ahead of you, but far enough away to not endanger you, an avalanche breaks loose. You see a pair of cross country skiers below directly in the path of the oncoming avalanche. What should you do at that moment?**
    a) Immediately turn and run for help so as to not lose time
    b) Watch where the avalanche takes the skiers and mark where the avalanche overtakes them. Then go for help or rescue.
    c) Go to the place where you last saw the skiers and begin working up the avalanche area from there looking for clues to where they are.
    d) Begin making an evacuation vehicle from a nearby tree then head down to the avalanche area and begin searching.

6. Which of the following is most likely to kill an avalanche victim the soonest?
   a) A broken arm that becomes gangrenous
   b) Hypothermia
   c) Asphyxiation
   d) Starvation

ANSWERS
1. c   2. e   3. d   4. e   5. c   6. c

CHAPTER 8

Bites and Stings

This chapter will train you on general issues related to preventing and treating bites and stings from the following land and marine creatures:

- Domesticated Animals
- Wild Animals
- Snakes
- Mosquitoes
- Spiders
- Ticks
- Hymenoptera
- Scorpions
- Jellyfish
- Stinging fish
- Sea snakes

Case 1

You and a friend are camping. You awake to roars and thumps outside your tent. Looking out the tent flap, you see your friend on the ground in the fetal position as a black bear knocks him around. You see potato chips scattered all over the campground.

1. What is the best approach to stopping the bear from attacking your friend?
2. Would your approach be different if you were in Canada and it was a Grizzly bear?

Case 2

You are camping with a friend when he comes running out of the woods being chased by several bees. After he has been running approximately one-fourth of a mile, the bees stop chasing him. Your friend comes to you with approximately 10 stings, several of which still contain the stinger with the sac attached. He does not have any breathing problems. He feels slightly dizzy from the whole event but does not appear sick.

1. What is the best way to remove the stingers from the wounds?
2. If you have an EpiPen®, should you use it on your friend?
3. Were these regular bees or Africanized Honey Bees?
4. Does he require evacuation from the site, or can you sit and watch him?

Case 3

A 24-year-old female has been swimming in the ocean when she notes the onset of an immediate stinging sensation on her arm and leg. Some 30 feet away you notice what appear to be a number of small "sails" floating on the water. On exam you notice a rash that has a "tentacle-like" appearance.

1. What should the immediate treatment be on the beach?
2. What is the cause?
3. What are the signs of severe envenomation one can see?

DOMESTICATED ANIMALS

General

The majority (80% - 90%) of domesticated animal bites are dog bites.

Cat bites account for 5% - 15% of domestic animal bites.

Victims of bites are often the pet owners or members of the pet owner's family.

Wilderness Care

Direct pressure should be used to stop bleeding.

Wounds that do not break the skin can be treated with ice and pain medications such as acetaminophen and ibuprofen.

The wound should be irrigated and cleaned as soon as possible, especially if the patient is greater than one hour from definitive medical care.

- ☐ Sterile water is not required, but the cleaner the water the better.
- ☐ Soap in the water increases the efficacy of cleaning and may decrease the potential for rabies.
- ☐ Irrigation should be done under high pressure.
- ☐ Dress the wound with a clean cloth.

Wound Infections

Infection is common with animal bites.

Bites are tetanus-prone wounds. Everyone should always ensure that their tetanus immunizations are up-to-date prior to entering the backcountry. Signs of tetanus include spastic paralysis, lockjaw, and sustained facial muscle spasms.

Rabies

Rabies is more commonly from bat, raccoon, and skunk bites than from dog bites in the United States.

In many parts of the world, dog bites are a very common transmitter of the rabies virus.

Good management of a wound can decrease the risk for rabies.

Domestic animal bites from an unknown or unvaccinated animal (typically dog or cat) should always be reported to animal control, and the victim should consider seeking further medical evaluation to assess the need for rabies treatment.

The Center for Disease Control (CDC) in the United States has a 24-hour helpline that can assist in determining the need to administer the rabies vaccine. The CDC can be contacted via the web at http://www.cdc.gov/rabies.

The disease pattern typically consists of fever, fatigue → agitation → paralysis, and coma → death.

Dog Bites

Prevention

- Never leave a child alone with a dog.
- Do not pet other people's dogs without permission.
- Do not kiss a dog.
- Do not lean over and pet a dog on the head.
- Do not physically separate fighting dogs; instead use a hose.
- Never take a bone or toy away from an unfamiliar dog.
- Do not approach a nursing dog.
- Teach injury prevention regarding dogs to children from an early age.
- Know the look of an angry dog and avoid interacting with dogs that are barking or growling and those that have teeth bared, ears flat, tail up, or hair on end.
- Never pet or step over a sleeping dog.

Treatment

- Immediate patient management and wound care should be performed as outlined above.
- Antibiotics should be considered for dog bites as these wounds are at higher risk for infection.

Cat Bites

Treatment

- Immediate patient management and wound care as outlined above.
- Cat bites have a higher infection rate in comparison to other domestic animals because they are more commonly puncture-type wounds. Any person with a significant cat bite should be evaluated for the need of antibiotics.

WILD ANIMALS

General

- The incidence of wild animal bites is difficult to ascertain as many minor wilderness bites and attacks are not reported.
- In Asia and Africa, thousands of people are killed yearly by attacks from lions, tigers, elephants, hippos, crocodiles, and snakes.
- In North America, large animals like bears and cougars kill very few people.
- In Yellowstone National Park, a visitor is more likely to be struck by lightning than to sustain serious injury from a large animal.
- A web site that tracks and compiles case reports of animal attacks is found at: http://attack.igorilla.com.

Prevention

- Animal behavior holds the key to prevention of most animal attacks.
- Aside from large carnivores, most animals do not attack humans unprovoked.
- The most common examples of human provocation of wild animals occur during time of animal capture or restraint.
- Even the shyest animal can inflict a life-threatening injury when cornered.
- If contact with an animal is likely or necessary, a detailed study of the animal's behaviors and cues should be undertaken to avoid mishap.

Treatment

- Wild animals that rarely carry rabies include rabbits, squirrels, chipmunks, opossums, rats, and mice.
- Wild animals that are at higher risk for carrying rabies include skunks, raccoons, foxes, and bats
- Treatment of wild animal attacks is similar to the treatment of a domestic animal attack.
- Evacuation should always be considered if a significant bite occurs from an animal that is at higher risk for rabies.

Bear Attacks

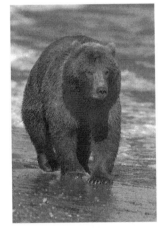

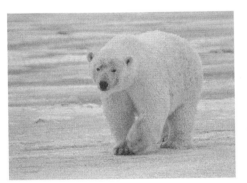

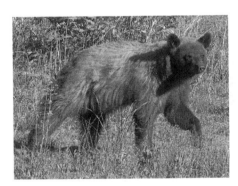

Figure 8.1. Black Bear
Photo by Michael Didier

Figure 8.2. Brown Bear
Photo courtesy of
www.naturespicsonline.com

Figure 8.3. Polar Bear
Photo courtesy
of www.naturespicsonline.com

Background

- North American bears include the brown (grizzly and Kodiak), American black, and polar bears. Brown bears vary in color from dark brown to blonde and can be distinguished from black bears due to their prominent shoulder hump and rounded face.
- Bears are fast (up to 40 mph) and large (140 to 1,400 pounds) with keen senses of smell and hearing.
- A bear's sight is equal to or less than a human's.
- Bear attacks are more common in the summer months because the bears are not hibernating and there are more visitors in the parks.
- The most common scenario ending in a brown bear attack is a sudden unexpected close encounter.
- Victims are rarely killed.

The wounds are described as a mauling, but the bear often inflicts the injuries and leaves without inflicting wounds to its maximum potential.

Situations that are more fatal include encroaching on a bear that is wounded, with a cub, or near a carcass.

In contrast to the brown bears, black bears rarely attack because of close encounters. Black female bears with cubs are more apt to flee an area if the human shows aggression.

Prevention

Make noise, such as talking, and allow the bears to move away from you.

Be cautious in environments where a bear may not be able to hear you such as near loud streams and in uneven terrain.

Avoid common bear areas such as streams with spawning fish, berry groves, and carcasses.

Camp in the open and cook your food away from your sleeping area.

Sleep upriver from your cooking site.

Maintain a clean camping site. Keep odorous products away from your sleeping gear.

Find a spot to hang your food at night above the ground where a bear cannot reach it.

If spotted by a bear, allow it to see you as human by stepping forward to allow the bear a full view of you.

If able to avoid an attack, retreat by waiting until the bear has left the area and move in the opposite direction.

Pepper spray may be useful if discharged directly at a charging bear's head when it is within thirty feet. Pepper spray is not to be used as mosquito repellant and pepper spray sprayed in a camp may actually serve as a bear attractant.

If you encounter a brown bear take the following actions:
- [ ] Do not look into the bear's eyes, as it is a sign of aggression.
- [ ] Do not make any sudden movements.
- [ ] Do not run.
- [ ] Do not act aggressively towards the bear.
- [ ] Just stand your ground but submissively.
- [ ] If attacked, get into the fetal position with your neck protected as they are "head oriented."

If you encounter a black bear, take the following actions:
- [ ] Yell, throw things, and act aggressively towards the bear as they usually will flee in response to aggression.
- [ ] If attacked – fight back as a black bear is likely viewing you prey
- [ ] If rolled onto your back, protect your face with your elbows.

Treatment

The possibility for significant injury is high.

All bear attack victims should be considered trauma victims and candidates for immediate evacuation.

Cougar Attacks

The North American cougar (mountain lion, puma) has come into contact with humans with increasing frequency.

Cougars are most commonly encountered in the western United States.

Cougars hunt by stealth, then pounce and break the victim's neck.

As with lions, cougars can potentially be scared off by the victim's aggressive behavior towards the animal. This is less likely in the case of a cougar with a cub or a wounded cougar.

When confronted by a cougar, you should face it, talk very loudly, and make yourself appear as a threat.

- Do not turn and run away from a cougar.
- If you have small children with you, pick them up as the cougar preferentially attacks children.
- If the cougar attacks, fight back using anything including rocks, sticks, bare fists, and fishing poles.

SNAKES

General

North America has two native types of poisonous snakes: the pit viper and the coral snake.

The overwhelming majority of envenomation in the U.S. come from pit vipers.

Annually, there are approximately 9,000 snakebites reported in the U.S.

From 1983 to 1998 there were only 10 deaths attributed to snake envenomation.

Pit Vipers

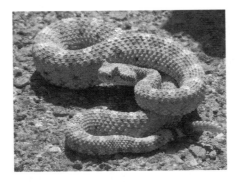

Figure 8.4 Diamond Back Rattle Snake – Pit Viper

Background

In the United States, pit vipers include the rattlesnake, copper head, and water moccasin (cotton mouth).

Pit vipers have a specific recognizable anatomy:
- [ ] Triangle shaped heads
- [ ] Catlike pupils
- [ ] Heat sensing pits between eyes and nose

Venom is dispersed from a tunnel in the fangs.

Approximately 25% of snakebites are "dry bites." This means that the snake injects no venom.

Pit viper venom can be hemotoxic (attacking tissue and blood) and/or neurotoxic (damaging or destroying nerve tissue).

In the U.S., pit viper venom is hemotoxic with the one exception being the Mojave rattler, which has neurotoxic venom. A bite from the Mojave rattler should prompt immediate evacuation and should be treated similar to a coral snake bite.

Each snake has a varying potency of its venom based on multiple factors:
- [ ] Emotional state of snake
- [ ] Species of snake as well as its size and age

- ☐ Time of year that the bite occurs
- ☐ Location of bite (more dangerous near vital organs)
- ☐ Size, age, and health of victim
- ☐ Depth of the bite
- ☐ Amount of venom injected (snakes can regulate the amount of venom released)

Clinical manifestations of pit viper envenomation

Severe burning at the bite site within minutes
Soft tissue swelling outward from the bite
Blood oozing from the bite
Bluish discoloration at the bite site and further down the limb
Nausea and vomiting
Weakness
Rubber, minty, or metallic taste in the mouth
Numbness of mouth and tongue
Uncontrollable muscle contractions
Increased heart and breathing rate
Difficulty breathing in severe cases
Shock

Treatment

Keep the victim calm and evacuate while minimizing physical activity.

Support the airway, breathing, and circulation while transporting.

Tight-fitting jewelry and clothing should be removed to avoid a tourniquet effect.

The swelling edge should be marked every 15 minutes for physicians and the hospital to assess the severity of the envenomation.

Immobilize and elevate the bitten extremity so that it is at the same level as the heart. Don't apply pressure.

Treatment with antivenin should be reserved for only at the hospital due to the potential serious complications, including severe allergic reaction or anaphylaxis.

Snake bite treatment has been plagued over the years with poor suggestions and bad information. The following is a list of things to avoid because they are either harmful to the patient or just do not work:

- ☐ The Sawyer Extractor™ may remove up to 20% to 30% of injected venom if applied within two to three minutes of the bite. However, there is a question whether the suction cup pressed against the skin causes further damage by exacerbating tissue necrosis. Further, there are no studies that show deceased morbidity or mortality through the use of the device.
- ☐ Avoid pressure immobilization. Simple immobilization is fine, but has no proven benefit.
- ☐ Electrotherapy should not used and can be harmful.
- ☐ Do not use ice as it may worsen local tissue damage.
- ☐ Do not attempt to try to catch or kill the offending snake. The recommendations for treating North American snakes' envenomation are the same for all types of snakes. Any attempts to capture the snake may result in additional envenomation and potentially another victim. Even a dead snake's jaw can clamp down and envenomate.
- ☐ Do not use aspirin, as it may worsen bleeding.
- ☐ Do not cut and suck on the wound as it may infect the wound with oral bacteria and it is ineffective at removing venom.

☐ Do not use alcohol on the wound or as an oral analgesic.
☐ Do not use a tight-fitting tourniquet that restricts blood flow.

Evacuation Guidelines

Victims of a pit viper bite should be promptly evacuated.

Coral Snake

Background

Coral snakes in the U.S. have a very distinct color banding pattern.
An easy way to remember the banding of the deadly coral snake is, "Red on black, venom lack; red on yellow, kill a fellow." This means that a red band adjacent to a yellow (not black) band means danger.
The bite of the coral snake typically involves a finger, toe, or fold of skin as its jaws are unable to open wide.
Coral snake venom is more potent than pit viper venom; however, envenomation usually takes up to twelve hours for a full effect.

Clinical manifestations of coral snake envenomation

Mild, transient pain at the time of the bite
No local swelling
Fang marks may be difficult to identify
Symptoms will often progress rapidly once they appear
Nausea and vomiting
Headache
Abdominal pain
Sweating and pale skin
Numbness and abnormal sensations
Drowsiness
Euphoria
Respiratory difficulties

Treatment

A more recent development for potentially inhibiting the absorption of the venom in the field is called the elapid wrap.
Wrap the area snugly with fabric in a way that will not impair blood flow.
Any type of fabric, including elastic bandages, works well.
Monitor for subsequent swelling that might make it too tight.
Otherwise, treatment and evacuation principles are the same as for envenomation with a pit viper.

Evacuation Guidelines

Victims of a coral snake bite should be promptly evacuated.

Snakes Worldwide

Worldwide, it is estimated there are a minimum of 1 to 2 million annual snakebite "incidences". This number includes bites by non-venomous species.

Of that number, roughly 50,000 to 100,000 bites result in fatalities worldwide. Many of the world's most venomous snakes have venoms that are very straightforward and 'easy' to treat effectively with the proper anti venoms.

There are some that cause a clinical explosion of problems for which anti venoms are not very effective.

Following is a list of the most dangerous and deadly snakes in the world using the potency of snake's venom, fatalities, and aggressiveness into account.

These bites must be treated aggressively, so it is essential to get to help quickly.

Pressure dressings and tourniquets are appropriate. Anti venom should be administered as soon as possible so immediate evacuation is essential.

It is important to know where these deadly snakes are found and to be aware of appropriate treatments and where hospitals would be located as a traveler goes to these various countries.

Black Mamba: The black mamba is found throughout most countries in Sub-Saharan Africa and is incredibly fast, traveling at speeds of up to 12 miles per hour. The Black Mamba is aggressive and territorial, characteristics not usually attributed to snakes. This snake is usually found in an olive green color – it's the inside of its mouth that is black. Its poison is a very fast acting neuro-toxin.

Russell Viper: This snake is found in Asia, throughout the Indian subcontinent, much of Southeast Asia, southern China and Taiwan. It is responsible for more human fatalities than any other venomous snake. It is a member of the big four venomous snakes in India, which are together responsible for nearly all Indian snakebite fatalities.

Egyptian Cobra: This is the most common cobra in Africa and is responsible for many deaths there. It typically makes its home in dry to moist savanna and semi-desert regions, with at least some water and vegetation.

Mozambique spitting cobra: This is a type of cobra, native to Africa. It is considered one of the most dangerous snakes in Africa, second only to the Mamba. It can spit its venom.

Australian brown snake: This is a deadly Australian snake. One 1/14,000 of an ounce of this vemon is enough to kill a person. It is the world's second most venomous land snake. Brown Snakes are very fast moving and highly aggressive. When agitated, they will hold their necks high, appearing in a somewhat upright S-shape. The snake will occasionally chase an aggressor and strike at it repeatedly.

Death Adder: This snake is native to Australia. It is one of the most venomous land snakes in Australia and the world.

MOSQUITOS

Prevention

Mosquitoes transmit many deadly diseases and have been shown to cause the deaths of 1 in 17 people alive today.

- Mosquitoes are attracted by CO_2, lactic acid, warm skin, and moisture. They also gravitate towards the smell of soap, detergents and perfume.
- Mosquitoes are most active at dusk, so staying indoors during that time will decrease contact.
- Choose a campsite that is high and away from standing water.
- Wear clothing with long sleeves and long socks with the pants tucked into the socks or boots.
- Wear clothing that is tightly woven, such as nylon, and is loose fitting so that a mosquito cannot bite through the clothing.
- Wear insect repellant on uncovered skin.
- DEET is the gold standard for insect repellants.
  - ☐ It is sold in formulations of 5%-35%.
  - ☐ Use formulations of 10% or less in children and avoid use altogether in infants under 6 months of age.
  - ☐ Use formulations of 30% to 35% in malaria-prone areas on adults.
  - ☐ Do not use sunscreens that contain DEET as sunscreens need to be used liberally and often, whereas DEET should be used less often.
  - ☐ When using both sunscreen and DEET, apply the sunscreen first then apply the DEET approximately 30 minutes later.
  - ☐ DEET may be applied to clothing but should be washed off as soon as repellent is no longer needed.
  - ☐ Oil of Lemon Eucalyptus is a plant-based substance and Picaridin (a chemical known also as Icaradin) are shown to be as effective as low concentrations of DEET in repelling mosquitoes. They have a pleasant fragrance and sprays containing these are far less likely to irritate the skin than DEET repellents.
- Permethrin is a naturally occurring compound with insecticidal and repellent properties that will stay on the material for weeks when properly applied.
- Apply Permethrin to clothing and bedding, especially mosquito netting. Do not apply directly to skin.
- If you are traveling to a location where you are unsure of the mosquito risk you can consult the CDC website: http://www.cdc.gov/travel/index.htm. This website is very helpful for comprehensive and up-to-date information on what immunizations (yellow fever) and prophylactic antibiotics (malaria) are recommended.
- In summary, current studies show Permethrin-treated clothing plus DEET repellent confers the best protection.

SPIDERS

Background

- Many spiders are venomous, but only a few of them are dangerous to humans.
  - ☐ Many spiders do not have enough venom to affect a human.
  - ☐ Many spiders do not have fangs large enough to penetrate human skin.
- Dangerous North American spiders include the black widow, brown recluse and hobo spider.

Black Widow

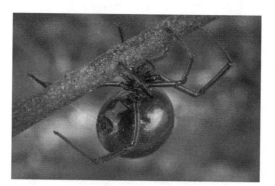

Figure 8.5 Black Widow Spider

Background

- The black widow is a female of the Lactrodectus species that is found worldwide.
- It is characterized by black shiny skin and a red mark on the belly (often an hour-glass shape).
- They make their homes in irregular webs in sheltered corners of vineyards, fields, and gardens. They can also be found under stones, logs, vegetation and trash heaps.

Clinical signs of a black widow bite

- A sharp pin prick is usually felt, although not always.
- Faint red bite marks may appear later.
- Muscle stiffness and cramps of the bitten limb may develop and will typically spread to involve the abdomen and chest.
- Additional symptoms include headache, chills, fever, heavy sweating, dizziness, nausea, vomiting, and severe abdominal pain.
- These symptoms occur within 30-60 minutes of the bite.
- Most black widow bites have excellent long-term outcomes.
- Short-term problems include high blood pressure, altered mental status, and abdominal pain.
- One study showed that only 25% of bite victims will go on to have the more serious symptoms. Very few humans die from black widow bites, and those who do are usually at the extremes of life or highly allergic.

Treatment

- Catch the spider, if possible, as even a smashed spider can be identified under the microscope of an experienced entomologist.
- Clean the bite with soap and water.
- Relieve pain with a cold compress and oral medications. Cold compresses will also reduce circulation to help slow the spread of the venom.
- *Latrodectus* antivenin may be used in the hospital in children and the elderly, but it is generally not used.

Evacuation Guidelines

The victim of a bite should be evacuated as soon as possible as envenomation can become very painful, and the patient may warrant more serious medical attention than can be given in the wilderness.

Brown Recluse

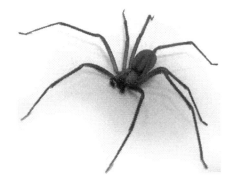

Figure 8.6 Brown Recluse Spider

Background

Loxosceles reclusa or the brown recluse is most commonly found in the southern states and up the Mississippi River Valley as far north as Wisconsin.

The brown recluse is nondescript and brown, although some will have a violin-shaped marking on the top front body portion.

Its habitat includes small sticky webs under rocks and woodpiles. The brown recluse also likes warm human habitats including homes, warehouses, and sheds.

Clinical signs of a brown recluse bite

The initial bite is usually painless. The victim is unaware that a bite even occurred until it becomes painful, red, itchy, and swollen two to eight hours after the bite.

The majority of bites remain localized, healing within three weeks without serious complication or medical intervention.

Additional symptoms include fever, weakness, vomiting, joint pain, and rash.

In more serious cases, the bite may cause significant local tissue damage, manifested in the following ways:

☐ It will have a white core surrounded by an erythematous patch of skin ending in a white, blue border. This can resemble a "bulls-eye" pattern.

☐ Within 24-48 hours, the central core will blister if the envenomation is more serious. This central core may continue to expand over a period of days to weeks if it is a more serious envenomation. Damage to the patient's skin and subcutaneous fat may occur leading to ulcerations.

Treatment

Catch the spider, if possible, to allow for identification.

Cleanse the bite with soap and water.

- Elevate the extremity and loosely immobilize it.
- Place a cold compress and give oral analgesics for pain control.
- The patient is in no immediate danger unless systemic signs begin appearing such as large patches of inflammation or blood in the urine.
- Hospital management is only necessary if systemic symptoms occur.

Evacuation Guidelines

- There is no need to evacuate the patient unless they develop systemic symptoms.

Hobo Spider

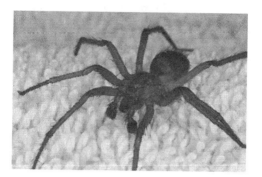

Figure 8.7. Hobo Spider
Photo by Dr. Lee Ostrom

Background

- Otherwise known as the *Tegenaria agrestis*, the Hobo Spider was introduced to the U.S. in the early 1900s from Europe and/or West Central Asia.
- It is now found throughout the Pacific Northwest U.S.
- It is a 10-15 mm brown spider with yellow-green tint on the dorsal abdomen and hairy legs.
- It builds funnel webs and is found near railroad tracks, under rocks, woodpiles, and in debris.

Clinical signs of a hobo spider bite

- Possible local tissue damage (similar to tissue damage from a brown recluse spider bite) at the bite site in 36 hours
- Headache, visual disturbances, hallucinations, weakness, and lethargy

Treatment

- Catch the spider, if possible, to allow for identification.
- Clean the bite with soap and water.
- Relieve pain with a cold compress and oral medications.
- Take victim to receive medical attention if signs of systemic reaction occur.

Evacuation Guidelines

There is no need to evacuate the patient unless they develop systemic symptoms.

TICKS

Background

Ticks transmit many diseases including Lyme Disease, Rocky Mountain spotted fever, and Colorado tick fever. Only the mosquito transmits more diseases worldwide than the tick.

Ticks are found in areas replete with weeds, shrubs, and trails.

They will often be found at forest boundaries where deer and other mammals reside.

Ticks will sit on whatever low-hanging shrub it can find with arms outstretched.

Once on a person, they may then take up to several hours to find a suitable spot to attach their mouth.

A tick will then feed on the blood of the host for an average of two to five days.

Prevention

Check clothing and exposed skin for ticks twice daily.

Tuck shirts into pants and pants into socks.

Wear smooth, close-woven, loose-fitting clothing.

Soak or spray clothing with Permethrin.

Wear DEET insect repellent.

Treatment

When a tick is removed in less than 48 hours patients rarely get Lyme disease. For this reason it is very important to check for ticks often and to remove them immediately upon discovery.

Tick removal:
- ☐ Use thin-tipped tweezers or forceps to grasp the tick as close to the skin surface as possible.
- ☐ Pull the tick straight upward with steady even pressure.
- ☐ Wash the bite with soap and water, then wash hands after the tick has been removed.

Watch for local infection and symptoms of tick-borne illness (3-30 days), especially headache, fever, and rash.

The **"DO NOTS"** of tick removal are the following:
- ☐ Do not use petroleum jelly.
- ☐ Do not use fingernail polish.
- ☐ Do not use rubbing alcohol.
- ☐ Do not use a hot match.
- ☐ Do not use gasoline.
- ☐ Do not grab the rear end of the tick. This expels contents and increases the chances of infection.
- ☐ Do not twist or jerk, as this will most likely cause incomplete removal of the tick.

Evacuation Guidelines

- Most patients with tick bites do not require evacuation, especially if the tick is removed within 24-48 hours.
- However, if the patient develops fever, headache, vomiting, rash, or other signs of systemic illness, the patient should be urgently evacuated

HYMENOPTERA

Background

- Hymenoptera is the order of insects that includes ants, bees, and wasps.
- Although there is great concern over snake bites, many more people die in the United States from bee, hornet, and wasp stings than from snake bites.
- One sting to an allergic person can be fatal in minutes to hours.
- Non-allergic victims may experience fatal toxicity if they sustain multiple stings.
- It takes between 500-1400 simultaneous stings to cause death by toxicity in the non-allergic patient.
- Multiple stings have become more of a concern in the U.S. since the Africanized Honey Bees ("Killer Bees") first arrived in 1990.

Clinical signs of hymenoptera sting

- The local reaction is the most common reaction. It consists of a small red patch that burns and itches with some pain.
- The generalized reaction consists of hives, swelling of lips and tongue, wheezing, abdominal cramps and diarrhea.
- Stings to the mouth and throat are more serious as they may cause airway swelling.
- Victims of multiple stings often experience vomiting, diarrhea, shortness of breath, lightheadedness and may even loss consciousness.

Prevention

- Do not wear any sweet-smelling fragrances often found in after-shaves and perfume. These often attract bees and other insects.
- Bees and wasps are attracted by rotten fruit and fruit syrups.
- Frequent cleaning of garbage areas and proper disposal of old fruit will decrease hymenoptera attraction.
- If an adult has had a full-fledged anaphylactic reaction, they should see an allergist for desensitization.
- A hymenoptera allergic patient should wear medical tags and carry an EpiPen® or equivalent device.

Treatment

- Scrape away the stinger in a horizontal fashion as it may continue to pump toxin into the wound.
  - ☐ Try not to grasp the stinger sac as that may pump more venom into the site.
  - ☐ However, if one is unable to remove the stinger in a horizontal fashion, removing it any way possible is more important rather than waiting.

- Wash the site with soap and water.
- Place a cold compress or ice on the site. This can ease the pain and swelling.
- Give oral pain medication as needed for pain relief.
- Seek immediate advanced medical attention if there is any shortness of breath, wheezing or other breathing concerns.

SCORPIONS

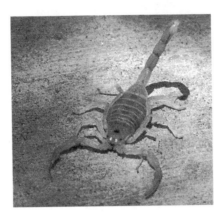

Figure 8.8 Bark Scorpion
Photo by Musides at
en.wikipedia

Background

- Scorpions are found in desert and semiarid climates between 50 degrees north and south latitude.
- Most scorpion stings are not lethal.
- Most scorpion stings result in only local pain and inflammation.
- In the U.S., the medically important scorpion is the Centruroides exilicauda or Bark Scorpion. This is found in the Southwestern U.S., primarily Arizona and New Mexico. The bark scorpion is long and slender and has a straw-colored yellow appearance with longitudinal stripes.
- In North America, more serious scorpion stings occur in Mexico.
- The bark scorpion can be lethal to infants and the elderly.
- The bark scorpion can be found under wood piles, stumps, firewood piles, trees and in a moist indoor environment under blankets, clothing, and in shoes.

Clinical signs of scorpion sting

- Scorpions may sting multiple times.
- Except for the bark scorpion, most sting symptoms are similar to hymenoptera stings.
- For the bark scorpion, the following conditions apply:
  - ☐ The sting causes local pain followed with numbness and tingling.
  - ☐ A toxin released at the time of the sting can cause muscle spasms and possibly changes in blood pressure and heart rate.

☐ Symptoms include paralysis, muscle spasms, breathing problems, vision problems, swallowing difficulty, and slurred speech.

Prevention

Check for scorpions in clothing and shake out shoes in areas where the scorpions are prevalent.
Do not place your hands or feet into unknown areas that you cannot look directly into.

Treatment

Clean the sting site with soap and water.
Place a cool compress for pain and swelling. Cooling the wound will facilitate your body's breakdown of the venom and reduce overall pain.
Oral pain medications can also be given if the patient does not have trouble breathing and the mental status is normal.
If the scorpion is identified as <u>not</u> being a bark scorpion, treat the sting as follows:
☐ Local treatment and monitoring similar to hymenoptera sting is all that is required.
☐ Evacuation is not mandated unless the patient develops significant symptoms.
■ If the scorpion is identified as a bark scorpion, treat the sting as follows:
☐ Evacuate as soon as possible as the patient may decompensate rapidly.
☐ The need for evacuation is more significant in children and the elderly.

MARINE ENVENOMATION

General

Marine creatures cause illness through a number of mechanisms, with the most common being through the injection of venom (envenomation).
Marine creatures of most common medical concern can be broken down into several groups:
☐ Jellyfish and Portuguese Man-O-War
☐ Stinging fish
☐ Sea snakes

Jellyfish and Portuguese Man-O-War

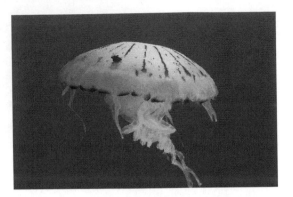

Figure 8.9 Jellyfish

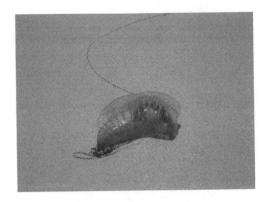

Figure 8.10 Man-O-War

Background

These ubiquitous marine creatures cause envenomation through their nematocyst stinging cells. When these cells contact skin, they essentially fire a venom-filled tube into the victim's skin.

The greater the number of nematocysts that contact the victim the greater the envenomation.

Envenomation can range from mild, which is the most common, to severe and life threatening.

Portuguese Man-O-War (Physalia species) and the Box Jellyfish (Chironex Fleckii) have the more toxic venoms encountered, with Chironex being the most deadly.

☐ The Box Jellyfish is located along northern Australia and the Indo-Pacific ocean.

☐ The Man-O-War is located in oceans across the world, generally in the warmer waters.

Clinical signs of jellyfish and Man-O-War envenomation

Mild envenomation

☐ Seen with most common jellyfish types.

☐ Skin irritation is the major symptom.

☐ The Man-O-War and the box jellyfish can cause envenomation from mild all the way to severe, depending on the degree of exposure to the tentacles.

Moderate envenomation

☐ Seen with larger envenomation such as with Portuguese Man-O-War.

☐ Skin symptoms occur with possible additional symptoms including the following:

   – Headache, vertigo, unsteady gait, numbness/tingling, paralysis, coma, and seizure

   – Difficulty breathing

   – Muscle pains, joint pains, and muscle spasms

   – Nausea, vomiting, and diarrhea

Severe envenomation

☐ Occurs most commonly due to significant box jellyfish exposure.

☐ Less commonly seen with the Portuguese Man-O-War but can occur with significant exposure.

☐ Though rare, deaths due to the Portuguese Man-O-War occur in the young, old, or those with severe allergic reaction on top of envenomation.

☐ Presents as more severe manifestations of moderate envenomation and can lead to loss of consciousness, convulsions, and even death.

Skin symptoms are the most common finding in Jellyfish envenomation. On contact with the tentacles the nematocysts discharge into the victim's skin and release the toxin.
- [ ] Numbness/tingling, itching, and "burning" or "stinging" pain can occur.
- [ ] Red-brown tentacle marks are noted.
- [ ] In severe cases, significant tissue damage can be seen.
- [ ] Systemic symptoms seen in more severe envenomation are as described above.

Treatment

Transport the victim to a safe place out of the water.

Rinse the wound with seawater. Do not use fresh water as it can cause the unfired nematocysts to fire and worsen the envenomation.

Remove tentacles with a gloved or otherwise protected hand.

Acetic acid 5% (vinegar) should be poured on the sting and tentacles as described below:
- [ ] It inactivates the nematocysts and toxin for jellyfish. Apply continuously until the pain resolves.
- [ ] It will not decrease the pain of the Chironex (box jellyfish) but will halt the envenomation.
- [ ] It may worsen the release of venom in Portuguese Man-O-War stings and should not be used on these stings or tentacles.

Isopropyl alcohol can be utilized if acetic acid is not available. However, this should not be used for Chironex (box jellyfish).

Once inactivated, the nematocysts should be removed.
- [ ] This is best done by applying shaving cream or baking soda and shaving off the nematocysts.
- [ ] If nothing else is available, make a paste of sand or mud and scrape it off with a straight edge.

In Man-O-War stings, hot water (45°C) may be utilized to effectively reduce pain **after** removal of nematocysts and irrigation of the sting area.

Cold packs may also decrease pain.

Because of the severe toxicity of the Chironex, its antivenom is often used in the pre-hospital environment in those areas where it is ubiquitous.

The "DO-NOTs" of Jellyfish and Man-O-War stings:
- [ ] Do not use freshwater to rinse the stings. Freshwater will cause more nematocysts to release.
- [ ] Do not rub the area as this will discharge more nematocysts.
- [ ] Do not use warm water or heat packs until the nematocysts have been shaved off. The heat may cause the nematocysts to discharge.
- [ ] Do not use acetic acid on Pacific Man-O-War stings.
- [ ] Do not use isopropyl alcohol for box jellyfish stings.

Evacuation Guidelines

Anyone with more than a minor envenomation and anyone with Chironex envenomation should be evacuated.

Stinging Fish

Background

"Stinging fish" includes many different fish with spines that include a venom apparatus.

The spines stick into the victim, break off, and venom is injected.

These creatures are found worldwide in salt water, with the catfish also found in inland fresh water.

Sea Urchins, although not "stinging fish," are similarly treated as they have envenomated spines.

Stinging fish includes the stonefish, lionfish, scorpionfish, stingrays, and catfish.

All have venom that is injected when one comes in contact with their spines or, in the case of a stingray, its tail.

All of these fish sting humans as a defensive measure, typically when accidentally grabbed or stepped on.

The toxin of the stonefish, scorpionfish, and lionfish is highly toxic causing muscle and nerve paralysis.

Stonefish venom is of such toxicity that it has been compared to the venom of the cobra.

Antivenom is available for treatment of stonefish poisoning and scorpionfish envenomation.

The extent of envenomation is dependent on the number of spines encountered and the type of fish.

Some parts of the venom of this group can be neutralized with heat.

Typically the venom-filled spine breaks off into the wound causing a dirty wound and retained foreign bodies, which lead to wound infection.

Sea urchin spines are brittle and break off easily in the flesh, resulting in both envenomation and a foreign body.

Clinical signs of stinging fish envenomation

Immediate and severe pain is the common hallmark of a sting from all members of this species.

Pain peaks in 30 - 90 minutes depending on the species and can last for hours to days if untreated.

Wound areas can develop bluish discoloration, redness, and swelling.

Stingray wounds also include a laceration component as the tail contains serrated teeth and it is stabbed into the victim with significant force.

Treatment

Clean the wound of any remaining debris as soon as possible and irrigate with warm/hot saline or potable water for initial wound care.

As opposed to jellyfish stings, warm/hot water <u>should</u> be used for stinging fish treatment.

- ☐ As soon as possible, the wound should be soaked in hot water at a temperature as high as tolerated; typically this is up to 113° F.
- ☐ The high temperature breaks down some of the venom and decreases pain.
- ☐ The soaks should be done for at least 30 minutes.
- ☐ Soaks may be repeated after one to two hours if pain returns.

Apply a sterile dressing and cover the wound with a loose bandage. This helps decrease the high risk of infection commonly seen in these injuries.

Limit swelling by keeping the wound elevated.

Control pain with oral medications as required.

Anti-venom is available in Australia for treatment of stonefish envenomation.

Anti-venom for scorpion fish stings is available in the U.S.

Evacuation Guidelines

Victims of a sting should be evacuated as soon as possible.

Sea Snake

Background

Sea snakes are found in tropical warm waters worldwide. The Persian Gulf and Southeast Asian Coasts are the areas of most frequent attacks.

Sea snakes are docile unless trapped or played with.

Almost all bites are due to stepping on, trapping, or otherwise mishandling the snakes.

Sea snakes have a variety of potent neurotoxins.

The venom of all varieties of sea snakes is similar.

Sea snake fangs are small and easily break off. Because of this, most sea snake bites cannot penetrate a wetsuit.

Symptoms may not develop for a few hours after a bite. However, if no symptoms occur in eight hours then the bite has not resulted in envenomation.

Clinical signs of sea snake envenomation

A sea snake bite is typically painless or at most a "pricking" sensation.

Symptoms typically begin within two to three hours of a bite.

Fatigue or anxiety is initially noted.

Muscle aches and stiffness are then noted, which then progresses to muscle spasms and eventual paralysis.

Speech and swallowing difficulty develop.

The more severe the envenomation is the more rapid the onset of symptoms will occur.

A lack of symptoms within eight hours of a "bite" means no envenomation has occurred.

Treatment

The involved limb should be immobilized. Movement can increase the toxicity of the poison.

☐ The immobilization wrap technique utilized for coral snakes can be used.

☐ Alternatively, a pressure dressing should be made of gauze placed directly over the fang marks and then covered with a circumferential pressure wrap such as an Ace bandage.

☐ This bandage should be 15 - 18cm wide and applied with enough pressure to inhibit venous, but not arterial blood flow. This can be ensured by checking the pulse beyond the wrapped area.

Ice should <u>not</u> be applied to bite.

Incision and suction of the bite site should <u>not</u> be performed.

Evacuation Guidelines

All victims of a sea snake bite should be evacuated immediately and considered for antivenom therapy if they display any signs of envenomation.

Twenty-five percent of victims bitten by venomous sea snakes die without antivenin.

QUESTIONS

1. True or False: When you accidentally encounter a black bear you should immediately get into the fetal position and protect your neck.

2. True or False: When confronted by a cougar you should face it and appear very noisy as if you are a threat to it.

3. True or False: Once a snake has been killed there is little risk is picking up a snake—in fact it is encouraged for identification.

4. For which one of the following snakes' bites would you consider wrapping the arm or leg with an obstruction wrap that does not occlude blood flow?
   a) Copper head
   b) Cotton mouth
   c) Diamondback rattlesnake
   d) Snake with red on black stripes
   e) Snake with red on yellow stripes

5. Which one of the following is an appropriate tick-removal technique?
   a) Light a match and burn the rear end of the tick
   b) Lather the tick and surrounding skin with Vaseline to require the tick to come up for air
   c) Pour alcohol over the tick as an irritant
   d) Remove gently with tweezers grasping as close to the skin as possible and pulling straight out
   e) Using tweezers, twist the tick so it will disengage its mouth and then pull straight out

6. Which one of the following is an appropriate field first aid measure for snake bite wound care?
   a) Cut down the track of the bite with a clean knife and suck on the cut
   b) Give aspirin for the pain
   c) Give antivenin early in the field if you have some in your aid kit
   d) Immobilize the bite at the level of the heart and require the patient to rest
   e) Place ice over the wound to decrease pain and swelling

7. A diver plays with a sea snake. He is not wearing gloves and notes a mild "pricking sensation" in his hand. Which one of the following is most appropriate for managing this patient?
   a) A venous obstructing tourniquet should be applied at the level of the wrist
   b) He can be observed at the site for eight hours and then evacuated if he starts to display symptoms
   c) The involved hand should have a pressure immobilization dressing applied
   d) Ice should be applied to the site to decrease any pain
   e) The area of potential bite should have incision and suction performed on it

8. **Which one of the following is correct regarding sea snakes?**
   a) Sea snakes are aggressive and will attack and bite if approached
   b) Sea snakes have a large fang apparatus that can easily penetrate a wetsuit
   c) Sea snakes do not have a toxic venom
   d) Sea snake bites always result in envenomation
   e) If symptoms do not develop eight hours after sea snake exposure, then the bite has not resulted in envenomation

9. **Which one of the following should be performed as first aid for stinging fish envenomation?**
   a) Acetic acid poured vigorously on the injury site
   b) Cold water immersion of the affected part
   c) Warm/hot water and immerse the affected part (false- make hot as patient will tolerate)
   d) Sodium hypochlorite (bleach) in a 1% solution

10. **A child inadvertently walks into several jellyfish in the shallow water. He develops "burning" pain over both lower legs where he touched the jellyfish. Which one of the following is most appropriate to treat this child?**
    a) Immersion in hot/warm water
    b) Rinsing with acetic acid (vinegar)
    c) Rinsing with hypochlorite (bleach) in a 1% solution
    d) Rubbing the area of the sting vigorously
    e) Wound rinsing with freshwater

11. **True or False: The stinger from a honeybee should be removed to prevent further toxin seepage, but one should not try to grasp the venom sack as that might pump more toxin into the wound site.**

12. **A bite from which spider would be cause for immediate evacuation?**
    a) Black widow
    b) Brown recluse
    c) Daddy long legs
    d) Hobo spider
    e) Tarantula

13. **True or False: A DEET-soaked wristband will repel mosquitoes from the wearer for hours at a time.**

14. **True or False: Most scorpion stings are poisonous and require immediate evacuation.**

ANSWERS
1. f 2. t 3. f 4. e 5. d 6. d 7. c 8. e 9. c 10. b 11. t 12. a 13. t 14. f

CHAPTER 9

Diving Medicine

In this chapter you will learn the potential complications of diving and treatment in the following areas:

Objectives:

- Review pathophysiology of diving medicine
- Review barotrauma
- Discuss care of overpressure syndromes
- Review decompression sickness (DCS)

GENERAL OVERVIEW

- Diving medicine is an expanding field as there are over 4 million recreational divers in the US alone.
- There are approximately 400,000 new dive certifications annually.
- There were 1,200 reported cases of decompression sickness (DCS) in 2004.

Types of Diving

- There are many types of diving, though SCUBA is the most common.
- Breath-hold diving
  - ☐ This is the simple holding of breath before diving under the water without breathing until resurfacing.
  - ☐ 2007 record: 704 feet (130 m)
- Scuba
  - ☐ Scuba is an acronym for Self Contained Underwater Breathing Apparatus.
  - ☐ Scuba diving is swimming (or occasionally walking) underwater wearing a breathing apparatus that allows the diver to breathe underwater at depth.
- Surface-supplied diving
  - ☐ This is also called hardhat diving.
  - ☐ With this type of diving, air is pumped in the suit from the surface.
- Saturation diving
  - ☐ Divers stay in living quarters at depth, thus they "saturate" with compressed gas.
  - ☐ They only decompress when they surface days later.
- ■ 1 ATA (Atmosphere Absolute) diving
  - ☐ This is diving with the air pressure only at 1 atmosphere (sea level).
  - ☐ This is diving in a submarine, including the one-man submarine.

Dysbarism

- Dysbarism is defined as problems that occur because of the physiologic effects of pressure.
- Dysbarism affects divers, compressed air workers, aviators, and astronauts amongst others.

Diving Physiology and Laws

- Pressure is a force-per-unit area or pressure = Force/Area
- Atmospheric pressure = 760mm (14.7 PSI) at sea level.
- Atmospheric pressure at sea level is also called 1 ATA (atmosphere absolute).
- Absolute pressure is total pressure (pressure from depth of water plus atmospheric pressure).
- Pressure gauges read zero at sea level; they have been adjusted to remove the effect of atmospheric pressure.
- Water
  - ☐ Each foot of sea water adds 0.445 PSI of pressure to the atmospheric 14.7 PSI at sea level.
  - ☐ Every 33 feet of sea water is 1 ATA.
  - ☐ At 33 feet of depth, the body experiences 2 ATA absolute pressure.
  - ☐ At 66 feet of depth, the body experiences 3 ATA absolute pressure.
- The change in pressure is linear with depth, but the greatest relative change is near the surface.
- The physiologic effects of pressure on the body are governed by two laws of physics.
  - ☐ Pascal's
    - – Pascal's law states pressure applied to any part of a fluid is transmitted equally through the fluid.
    - – Most of the human body is a liquid and thus follows Pascal's law.
  - ☐ Boyle's
    - – Boyle's law states that the pressure of a gas is inversely related to its volume.
    - – As pressure increases with descent, the volume of a gas bubble decreases, and as pressure decreases with ascent, the volume of that gas bubble increases.
    - – Air-containing spaces act according to Boyle's law. This predominantly means the lungs, middle ear, sinuses and GI tract.

Pressure in air-filled spaces of body is in equilibrium with environment and other air-filled spaces.
- ☐ These spaces remain in equilibrium with the environmental pressure unless the passageway that allows equilibrium with the rest of the environment becomes obstructed.
- ☐ If this occurs, disequilibrium develops and barotrauma can result.

Divers Alert Network (DAN)

The definitive go-to network for dive medicine information as well as consults on dive injuries.
1-919-684-9111 available 24/7/365. They will accept collect calls. If out of the USA check for the DAN number.

DECOMPRESSION SICKNESS (DCS)

Originally known as "Caissons" disease or "the bends" because it was first described in bridge builders working in underwater caissons, which had compressed air pumped into them to keep the water out for construction.

DCS has a reported Incidence of 1:7,500 dives.

It is caused by the formation of inert gas bubbles in blood as gas dissolved in solution by high-partial pressure comes out of solution on exposure to lower pressures.

Henry's law is the physics law that concerns the development of DCS.
- ☐ Henry's law states that the amount of inert gas that goes into and out of solution is based on the pressure (depth) and time of exposure.
- ☐ Thus, the deeper and longer one dives, the more inert gas that goes into solution and the more time that is required for it to come out of solution safely.

DCS is a multi-system disorder caused by a rapid decrease in atmospheric pressure.

By ascending faster than the gas can safely come out of solution into the lungs, the excess gas rapidly comes out of solution, forming bubbles in the tissue and blood.

In addition to the mechanical (ischemic) effects of the bubbles, they also activate the immune system, causing further injury through diffuse inflammation.

■ DCS onset occurs after surfacing.
- ☐ This often occurs within an hour (not as fast as AGE) and the majority of the DCS cases (95%) are seen within 6 hours.
- ☐ In rare cases it may not be noted for 24 - 48hrs.

CNS, cutaneous, pulmonary and musculoskeletal symptoms may be seen.

DCS was previously described as type I, II and III but it is now described as Musculoskeletal DCS, Cutaneous DCS, Systemic DCS or Neurological DCS.

DCS Symptoms

- ☐ Joint pain
- ☐ Paresthesias (numbness and tingling)
- ☐ Dysesthesias (unpleasant sense of touch)
- ☐ Weakness to paralysis
- ☐ Headache
- ☐ Confusion
- ☐ Skin itching

☐ Skin mottling (cutis marmorata)
☐ Dyspnea (shortness of breath)
☐ Coma

Musculoskeletal DCS

Can involve any joint, though shoulders and elbows are the most common.

Movement worsens the pain, which makes it difficult to differentiate from other musculoskeletal causes based on history or exam.

Some exam findings that suggest DCS are relieved of pain in a joint by inflating a BP cuff to over 200mm Hg over the joint, or an increase in pain seen by "milking" the muscle towards the joint.

CNS DCS

The spinal cord is most commonly involved.

Cerebral symptoms can occur but are much more common with AGE.

The initial symptom may start as back pain then progresses to paresthesias/paralysis.

Symptoms can be dynamic and not follow nerve pathways because the bubbles come out of solution in multiple areas.

Systemic DCS/ Pulmonary DCS "the chokes"

This is due to formation or passage of bubbles into the pulmonary system, which causes an effect of multiple "bubble" pulmonary emboli.

The initial symptoms are chest pain, cough with increasing pulmonary congestion and possible cardiovascular collapse.

Skin DCS

Itching is the most common skin manifestation of DCS and does not require recompression.

Mottling (cutis marmorata), however, is a forerunner of more severe DCS and recompression should occur.

DCS Treatment

The primary treatment is recompression as soon as possible.

High-flow oxygen should be given if available.

■ The following treatment adjuncts are not recommended:
☐ Aspirin and Ibuprofen and Aleve were routinely used for DCS in the past but are no longer recommended.
☐ Steroids are also not recommended for use in DCS treatment.

DCS prevention

Dehydration is to be avoided.

Dive computers or dive tables should be correctly utilized.

Flying after diving should be delayed for 12-24 hours or more after surfacing depending on the depth and duration of the dives.

Risk factors for DCS include:

- Obesity
- Smoking
- Flying after diving
- Patent Foramen Ovale (Opening in the upper chambers of the heart)

BAROTRAUMA

- Barotrauma = tissue damage as a result of pressure disequilibrium.
- The most common medical problems in diving are related to barotrauma.

Mask Squeeze

- Mask-pressure equilibrium is maintained by nasal exhalation.
- Failure to exhale into the mask results in a negative mask pressure as the diver descends due to shrinkage of the gas volume. This creates a vacuum that pulls the face into the mask.
- This results in skin bruising and conjunctival (eye) hemorrhage.

Ear Squeeze (Barotitis Media)

- This is by far the most common diving medical problem, with at least 40% of divers affected.
- At a depth of just 2.5 (1 m), a 60mm pressure gradient is developed across the middle ear with slight pain noted at this point.
- At a depth of 4 ft, (1m) a 90mm pressure gradient exists.
  - □ This results in collapse of the Eustachian tube and an inability to maintain equilibrium within the middle ear.
  - □ At this pressure, gradient attempts to equalize by Valsalva maneuver may not succeed.
- At 100 - 400mm gradient, 4 - 17 ft, (1 – 5 m), the tympanic membrane (TM) ruptures.
  - □ When this occurs, underwater serum and water are pulled into the middle ear.
  - □ If cold water enters the middle ear transient, vertigo, nausea and or vomiting may occur.
- Ear squeeze is preventable; this is done by "clearing" ears on water entry.
- It is especially likely to develop if there is any Eustachian tube dysfunction from a URI, allergies, or smoking. All these both predispose to ear squeeze as well as it make it difficult to clear the ears.
- Ear squeeze is treated with decongestants and analgesics as well as an antihistamine if an allergic component exists.
  - □ Afrin-type nasal sprays can be beneficial in helping to prevent ear squeeze if taken before diving in those with nasal congestion.
  - □ Eustachian tube "clearing" can be done as often as required by performing a gentle Valsalva (forceful attempted exhaling against a closed mouth) or Frenzel (pinching nose and swallowing) maneuver.
  - □ It is best to attempt these any time congestion is noted and as often as needed rather than trying to descend further without attempting.
  - □ If ear squeeze develops, one should not dive until it has resolved.
  - □ Systemic antibiotics are only given for a perforated TM.

☐ Topical antibiotics should be carefully chosen if the TM is perforated, as many are ototoxic.

Sinus Squeeze (Barosinusitis)

This is caused by the same basic mechanism as sinus squeeze.

As one descends, the air pocket in the sinus shrinks if it has no communication with the oropharynx.

This causes a vacuum in the sinus, which results in vacuum damage to the sinus wall with resultant pain and bleeding into the sinus.

The process is reversed on ascent, resulting in a "reverse sinus squeeze."

Treatment for this is the same as that for barotitis media.

Inner Ear Window Rupture

Two windows are at the opening to the inner ear from the middle ear. These can rupture.

This is a form of inner ear barotrauma occurring from a forceful Valsalva or rapid descent

Results in inner ear bleeding, oval or round window tear

Symptoms are roaring tinnitus, vertigo, hearing loss and ear fullness.

Similar to other types of inner ear insult, one can also have associated nausea, vomiting, vertigo, and ataxia (unstable gait).

It is usually associated with barotitis media, as the rupture occurs when trying to forcefully "clear" with a Valsalva maneuver.

Hearing loss is present.

Initial therapy is bed rest, with the head at 30°as well as referral for ENT evaluation.

An important consideration is to differentiate window rupture from inner ear DCS, as the treatments are significantly different. Window rupture occurs on the descent, usually with forceful Valsalva attempts.

Inner ear DCS occurs after ascent. If the diagnosis is uncertain, obtain help from the Diver's Alert Network (DAN).

PULMONARY OVERPRESSURE SYNDROME

The various forms of pulmonary overpressure syndromes (POPS) result from the expansion of gas trapped in lungs.

On ascent, the trapped gas expands and ruptures the tiny alveoli escaping into the local tissues or the systemic circulation.

This occurs from rapid uncontrolled ascent to the surface without sufficient exhalation to allow the gas escape.

Shallow depths are the most dangerous due to the greater relative percentage of pressure change.

A sudden 80 mm alveolar difference (which could occur with as little as 3 – 4 ft change in shallow depth) can force air across alveolar-capillary membrane.

Deaths have occurred from 6 ft (2 m) depth.

POPS can lead to arterial gas embolism (AGE).

Mediastinal Emphysema (Air in the Area Around the Heart)

Also called pneumomediastinum

This is the most common type of POPS.

Symptoms:
- ☐ Pain under the sternum
- ☐ Hoarseness of the voice
- ☐ Shortness of breath
- ☐ Neck pain

X-rays at a hospital are needed to confirm the diagnosis.

Treatment is to avoid further pressurization
- ☐ Placement of a chest tube is not required.

Arterial Gas Embolism (AGE)

This is the most feared complication of POPS.

It results from alveolar/vascular wall rupture with air bubbles entering the pulmonary veins.
- ☐ These bubbles then migrate into the left ventricle, aorta, and arterial system.
- ☐ The bubbles then shower distally and can obstruct blood flow in the distal vessels.
- ☐ They can affect both coronary and cerebral vessels.
- ☐ If the coronary (heart) vessels are involved, and MI (heart attack) can occur.
- ☐ If the cerebral (brain) vessels are affected, then a stroke can result. The brain symptoms that occur depend on where the air causes obstruction, thus they can be myriad, multi-focal and deadly.

AGE symptoms occur almost immediately on surfacing. They usually occur in less than two minutes but may take up to ten minutes to appear.

They will not occur later, as pulmonary pressures return to normal as soon as surface breathing starts.

Symptoms in a diver occurring immediately upon surfacing are due to AGE until proven otherwise.

Treatment for AGE is immediate recompression.
- ☐ Nothing should delay this.
- ☐ Give oxygen and supportive care.
- ☐ Maintain the patient in a supine position.
- ☐ Tilting the patient back and on the side is NOT recommended. Historically, these positions were recommended, but this recommendation has changed.
- ☐ AGE treatment with recompression may be effective even if the recompression cannot be performed until up to 24 hours later.
- ☐ Recompression reduces bubble volume, allowing return of blood flow to the obstructed areas.
- ☐ Even neurological symptoms that have resolved should still be treated with recompression.

If a patient requires air evacuation to reach treatment, the aircraft should fly no more than 500 ft. (125m) above ground level.

Recompression will occur in a hyperbaric chamber according to a number of protocols developed specifically for treatment of AGE.

DAN can provide the location of the nearest hyperbaric chamber if required.

HYPERBARIC GAS MEDICAL PROBLEMS

Inert Gas Narcosis

It is also known as "the narcs" or the "rapture of the deep."

It is primarily seen with nitrogen exposure (nitrogen narcosis) but can occur with many inert gases.

It results from the anesthetic effect of the inert gases that the diver is breathing.

As the partial pressure of that gas increases, cellular membranes are affected by the absorption of these inert gases into their lipid (fat) component.

☐ The greater the lipid solubility, the more narcotic potency of that gas.

☐ NO_2 >> N_2 >>>>>> He (helium)

☐ Helium is essentially non-narcotic and therefore commonly used as a mixed gas for diving.

Nitrogen narcosis is the most common due to divers breathing compressed air, which is 79% nitrogen.

☐ It begins around 70 - 100 ft (25 – 30m) and by 150 ft (50m) intoxication sets in.

☐ By 250 ft, (80m) auditory and visual hallucinations occur.

☐ At 400 ft, (125m) loss of consciousness occurs.

☐ Sport divers should dive at less than 100 ft (33m) to avoid this complication.

Oxygen Toxicity

Oxygen causes toxicity to the lungs and CNS (central nervous system) through several different mechanisms.

Oxygen toxicity is primarily a concern for those divers who dive on special mixtures other than compressed air.

Oxygen toxicity is primarily a concern for the deep divers and for those divers who are breathing mixtures that contain more than regular compressed air (21% oxygen).

Pulmonary Toxicity

This results primarily from the formation of oxygen-free radicals and the resultant tissue damage.

This requires one to breathe high oxygen concentrations for long periods of time.

Pulmonary toxicity can occur at sea level from prolonged exposure to high oxygen concentrations.

Pulmonary toxicity is also known as the "Smith effect."

Time limit before it starts to occur

☐ 0.5 ATA – indefinitely

☐ 1 ATA – 20 hours (~breathing compressed air at 130 ft (40m) = 0.21 x 5 atmospheres)

☐ 2 ATA – 6 hours

Symptoms of pulmonary toxicity

☐ Substernal chest discomfort on inhalation that progresses to burning pain

☐ Persistent coughing

☐ Prolonged toxicity can lead to a loss of vital lung capacity

CNS toxicity

Results primarily from oxidation of enzyme systems

- CNS toxicity will only occur with hyperbaric oxygen exposure.
- CNS oxygen toxicity is also called the "Bert Effect" after the first individuals to describe them in the late 1800s.
- CNS Toxicity requires much higher oxygen exposure than that causing pulmonary toxicity and occurs at 2.0 ATA or higher oxygen exposure.
- Symptoms of CNS toxicity
  - ☐ The earliest symptoms are typically twitching of the facial muscles and small muscles of the hands.
  - ☐ Apprehension
  - ☐ Seizures – these are not inherently dangerous, unless you drown.

QUESTIONS

1. A friend you are diving with for some reason rapidly ascends. On the surface she complains of chest pain, shortness of breath, neck pain and her voice is hoarse. She likely had developed:
   a) POPs syndrome with mediastinal air
   b) Gas narcosis
   c) Decompression sickness

2. A friend you are diving with ascends more rapidly then she should have. She complains of muscle pain, headache, and unpleasant sense of touch to the skin, tingling and confusion. She likely has developed:
   a) POPs syndrome with mediastinal air
   b) Gas narcosis
   c) Decompression sickness

3. You and a friend are diving around below 100 feet (30m). She begins to act strangely and then appears to have a small seizure. She most likely has?
   a) POPs syndrome with mediastinal air
   b) Gas narcosis
   c) Decompression sickness

ANSWERS
1. a 2. c 3. b

CHAPTER 10

Drowning and Water Safety

This chapter will train you to treat conditions caused by accidental drowning and methods to prevent this type of injury, according to the following criteria.

Objectives:

- Be able to define the basic terms of drowning, the drowning process, and survival
- Be able to describe the mechanism of shallow water blackout
- Be able to describe the basic pathophysiology of the drowning process
- Be able to describe the effects of drowning on the pulmonary system
- To demonstrate the initial management of a victim of a drowning in the wilderness setting
- Be able to describe which patients require evacuation to a medical setting
- Be able to describe methods to prevent drowning

Case 1

An eighteen-year-old male falls out of a raft in a class IV rapid and is repeatedly pulled under the water as he fights his way through the rapids. He is pulled out of the water on the shore and is awake and alert. He is coughing vigorously and complains of shortness of breath and a full sensation in his chest. His past medical history is unremarkable. Vital signs: P = 108, RR = 26.
Physical examination is remarkable for obvious respiratory distress with retractions and rales throughout his lungs. The remainder of his examination is normal.

1. What is the next step in the management of this patient?
2. Are there any other vital signs you would be interested in obtaining for this patient, if possible?
3. Are there any medications you could treat him with that you would normally carry with you?
4. Does he require evacuation to a hospital or can he stay in the backcountry with observation?

Case 2

You are camping by a lake and hear a cry for help. A father is holding his two-year-old son who is crying. According to the father, he was in the shallow water of the lake with his child and he turned his head away for "just a couple of seconds." When he turned back, he noticed his son was under the water and not moving. He immediately grabbed his son who started crying. There was no color change. The child is alert and crying. Vital signs: P=108, RR=20. Physical exam is normal to include normal respiratory efforts and a normal pulmonary exam.

1. What is your next step in the management of this child?
2. Are there any other vital signs you would be interested in obtaining?
3. Does this child require evacuation to a hospital or can he stay at the campsite with observation?
4. If you elect to observe this child, what is the time interval you should observe him?

BACKGROUND

Terminology

Drowning: A process resulting in primary respiratory impairment from submersion / immersion in a liquid medium. The victim may live or die during or after this process. The outcomes are classified as death, morbidity, and no morbidity.

The Drowning Process: A continuum that begins when the victim's airway lies below the surface of liquid, usually water, preventing the victim from breathing air. A victim may be rescued during the drowning process and may not require intervention or may receive appropriate resuscitative measure. In this case, the drowning process is interrupted. However, if the victim is not ventilated soon enough or does not start to breathe on his own, circulatory arrest will ensue, and in the absence of effective resuscitative efforts, multiple organ dysfunction and death will result.

Drowned: refers to a person who dies from drowning

Near drowning: It is the consensus of the International Liaison Committee on Resuscitation (ILCOR) that the term near drowning no longer be used. The term refers to survival for at least 24 hours after a successful rescue from a submersion episode. This usage has led to uncertainty about the meaning of the term, because it has implied certain recovery in many instances, which is not always the case. Furthermore, when the term is translated from English into other languages, the meaning is confusing and imprecise.

Survival: Indicates that the victim remained alive after the acute event and any acute or subacute sequelae.

Immersion: To be covered in water. For drowning to occur, at least the face and airway are immersed.

Submersion: During submersion, the entire body, including the airway, is under water.

Dry vs. Wet Drowning : The ILCOR recommends that these terms be abandoned.

The terms wet and dry have been used to classify as those who aspirate liquid into their lungs (wet) and those who do not (dry). Frequently it is not possible to determine at the scene whether or not water was aspirated, particularly when the amount of water is small.

Freshwater vs. Saltwater Drowning

At one time, based on animal studies, it was believed that different pathologic pathways existed between drowning in fresh water and salt water.

Freshwater drowning: It was theorized that with freshwater drowning, the aspirated water would be hypotonic and would rapidly pass through the lungs and go into the intravascular compartment. This would create fluid overload and a dilutional effect on serum electrolytes.

Saltwater aspiration: It was theorized that the hypertonic saltwater would cause fluid to be drawn into the alveoli, thus creating massive pulmonary edema and hypertonic serum.

In reality, patients who survive a drowning incident do not aspirate enough volume to cause hemodilution or electrolyte changes

☐ The one exception is the Dead Sea, which is extremely hypertonic. In surviving victims, significant effects on serum calcium and magnesium have been observed.

Shallow Water Blackout

A special cause of drowning that occurs in people who hyperventilate before entering the water for an underwater swim.

Hyperventilation significantly reduces the carbon dioxide level without increasing oxygen storage.

The vigorous underwater activity uses the available oxygen, causing hypoxemia (low blood oxygen) but before sufficient CO_2 accumulates to provide a stimulus to return to the surface. The patient loses consciousness due to the low oxygen and sustains a drowning event.

Epidemiology

In many areas of the world, drowning is a leading cause of death, especially among young children.

According to the World Health Organization, more than 500,000 deaths each year are due to drowning. Since all cases of fatal drowning are not classified as such even for high-income countries, this number probably underestimates the real figures.

Drowning is second only to motor vehicle accidents as the most common cause of accidental death in the United States

Annually in the U.S., there are an estimated 3,880 fatal drownings.

Drowning mainly kills the young.

- ☐ 64 percent of all victims are under age 30
- ☐ 26 percent of all victims are under age 5
- ☐ There is a bimodal age distribution in the young with large numbers of deaths in children age 4 and younger with the second larger increase in adolescents ages 15 to 24.

Freshwater drowning, especially in pools, is more common than saltwater drowning. This includes coastal areas.

Risk factors:

- ☐ Age
  - – Children ages 1 - 4 have the highest drowning rate.
  - – Among children ages 1 - 14, drowning is the second leading cause of unintentional injury death behind motor vehicle accidents in the United States.
  - – The risk of drowning for males increases at age 15 and remains elevated through age 24 years.
- ☐ Location - Victims of different ages drown in different locations.
  - – For children ages 4 and under, home swimming pools, bathtubs, buckets pose the greatest risk.
  - – Over half of the fatal and non-fatal drownings in adolescents occur in natural water settings, such as lakes, rivers, and oceans.
- ☐ Gender – Nearly 80% of people who die from drowning are male
- ☐ Drugs - Alcohol, in particular, is involved in half of adolescent and adult deaths associated with water recreation
- ☐ Trauma (secondary to dives, falls, and horseplay)
- ☐ Failure to wear a personal floatation device (PFD) - Most boating deaths are caused by drowning with 88% of the victims not wearing PFDs

PATHOPHYSIOLOGY

General

The basic pathophysiology of submersion injury is respiratory failure with hypoxemia and resultant cardiac death and neurologic injury.

Older victims who are not immediately unconscious may initially panic and struggle in the water.

- ☐ They will hold their breath or hyperventilate and try to stay above the water surface.
- ☐ Breath holding will occur.
- ☐ Eventually, a breaking point is reached and the body involuntarily breathes, even if the victim is under water. This point is determined by the both the blood levels of oxygen and of carbon dioxide.
- ☐ At the point of involuntary breathing, aspiration and vomiting occur with an impact on at least the pulmonary system.

Regardless of the drowning (wet, dry, fresh water, or salt water), the patient will have a similar outcome.

Organ System Effects

Pulmonary

The lung is the primary organ of injury.

Aspirated water the blood vessels in the lung to constrict that cases the blood pressure in the lung to raise.

Aspirated water also has a significant effect on lung tissue due to the washing out and destruction of surfactant.

All of these effects lead to significant breathing problems that can be mild to severe depending on the extent of the pulmonary injury.

Clinical signs and symptoms:

- ☐ Shortness of breath
- ☐ Air hunger
- ☐ Cough
- ☐ Wheezing

Cardiovascular

Cardiac arrhythmias (irregular heart beat) are common and significant in drowning incidents. However, these are usually secondary to the low blood oxygen levels.

Central Nervous System

12 to 27 percent of drowning victims sustain neurologic damage.

The best predictor of long-term neurological outcome is a normal or rapidly improving mental status during the first 24 hours after the drowning incident.

Insults to the CNS usually result from the hypoxia and/or trauma to the brain or spinal cord.

If the patient has an altered mental status, appropriate evaluation must look for CNS trauma as a source and one should not just ascribe the symptoms to the hypoxia.

Be concerned for cervical spine injuries when victims have been diving into pools or waters of unknown depth.

Cold Water Drowning

Water conducts heat 25 - 30 times better than of air. Children are at greatest risk of hypothermia associated with cold water drowning because of their larger body surface area.

Cold-water submersion results in rapidly induced hypothermia. The body's initial physiologic response to this insult is a fast heart rate and a fast breathing rate.

Hypothermia leads to muscle fatigue and poor judgment, decreasing the ability to self-rescue.

Theories of how neuroprotective hypothermia may occur prior to irreversible hypoxia include:

☐ The diving reflex, which includes a slow heart rate and the cessation of breathing.

☐ A combination of external skin exposure, icy water aspiration, and ingestion enabling a rapid core temperature drop.

☐ Through these mechanisms, it is postulated that hypothermia decreases cellular metabolism and may limit reperfusion injuries after resuscitation, especially in children.

However, most hypothermic drowning victims are cold from prolonged exposure and are simply dead.

TREATMENT

Rapid but cautious rescue so that the rescuers do not become victims.

The gold standard is immediate and aggressive initiation of ventilation and oxygenation.

Always consider coexistent trauma and institute spinal protections if there is any concern.

If possible, measure blood oxygenation with a pulse oximeter.

Administer oxygen if available.

CPR should be started on any patient with even a remote possibility of success.

☐ Prompt initiation of rescue breathing or positive pressure ventilation increases survival.

☐ Drowning victims with only respiratory arrest usually respond after a few rescue breaths.

☐ Interestingly, the Europeans Resuscitation Council recommends five initial rescue breaths instead of two (as recommended by the American Heart Association) because the initial ventilations can be more difficult to achieve in drowning victims.

☐ If there is no response to the initial rescue breaths, the victims should be assumed to be in cardiac arrest and be taken as quickly as possible to dry land where effective CPR can be initiated.

☐ Victims of cold-water submersion should ideally be warmed to approximately 90°F before the resuscitation is terminated.

☐ Victims of warm water submersion or those who are normothermic and have CPR ongoing for 20 to 30 minutes without success may have CPR terminated.

There are no special drainage procedures to "empty" water out of the lungs or stomach.

The Heimlich maneuver at one time was recommended by the American Red Cross and AHA. However, this technique is no longer recommended.

If the person in unconscious but breathing, the recovery position should be used.

Bronchospasm may be treated with beta agonists, such as albuterol.

The Asymptomatic Patient

In the wilderness, there will be drowning "events" when there is a question of whether an individual actually aspirated any water or had any significant hypoxia before being rescued.
- These patients may have some initial coughing as soon as being brought out of the water but will have no cough or respiratory complaints after the initial few minutes.
- They will have a normal respiratory rate and normal lung sounds exam if you listen by placing your ear on their chest.

These patients can be observed without evacuation for a period of six hours.

After six hours, if the patient still has no respiratory complaints, no cough, and continues to have a normal pulmonary exam then they can continue on with the trip.

If they develop any respiratory complaints, develop an abnormal exam or vital signs then they should be evacuated.

PROGNOSIS

Statistics on survival and the incidence of severe neurological deficits after a drowning event are difficult to interpret.

Unfavorable prognostic factors:
- Age 3 and younger
- Estimated submersion/ immersion time longer than five minutes
- No resuscitation attempts for at least 10 minutes after rescue
- Patient in a coma on ED admission
- Arterial blood gas pH 7.1 or less

With two or less of these factors present, there is a 90 percent chance of recovery.

The presence of three or more of these factors reduces the chance of survival to less than 5%.

EVACUATION GUIDELINES

Evacuate the following patients
- Those who suffered a loss of consciousness
- Any patient who required resuscitation, even if it was just rescue breathing
- Those who have any difficulty breathing, persistent cough or complaints of air hunger
- Those patients with tachypnea or an abnormal lung examination
- Those patients with hypoxemia, if you have a pulse oximeter available

Those patients who are asymptomatic with no respiratory distress may be observed for a period of at least six hours for development of new respiratory symptoms. If they are asymptomatic for this entire period, then they do not require evacuation.

PREVENTION

- Prevention is more important than any action one can take after a submersion incident has occurred.
- Alcohol should be avoided when participating in or supervising water activities.
- Everyone on a boat should always wear approved personal flotation devices that will support the person's head above water, even if the person becomes unconscious.
- Camp far enough away from water so that people, especially children, do not accidentally wander into the water.
- Anyone who works on or near the water should have swimming, rescue, and life-saving skills.
- Young children should always be supervised when around water.
  - ☐ A one-minute phone call or other distraction is all it takes for a child to become submerged.
  - ☐ Toddlers have drowned in toilets and small buckets of water.
  - ☐ Toddlers have drowned in bathtubs when left alone with older siblings to watch them without adult supervision.
- Patients with seizure disorders should always be supervised if swimming and should probably bathe in showers.
- Swimming pools:
  - ☐ These should be completely enclosed by a 5-foot fence with self-closing and self-latching locks.
  - ☐ This fence should also separate the pool from the house. This means that the pool should not be directly open to the back door of the house.
  - ☐ Appropriate life-saving equipment such as a pole to pull people to the side and personal flotation devices should be near the pool.
  - ☐ Owners of swimming pools should be trained in CPR.
  - ☐ Children whose families have a pool should take swimming lessons early.

QUESTIONS

1. **Which one of the following is the mechanism behind shallow water blackout?**
   a) Hyperventilation results in an increased blood oxygen level, causing one to lose the drive to surface to breathe
   b) Hyperventilation results in an increased blood carbon dioxide level, causing one to lose the drive to surface to breathe
   c) The lowered carbon dioxide level from hyperventilation causes one to seize and lose consciousness under the water
   d) The oxygen level in the blood drops too low before one has the drive to surface to breathe
   e) Vigorous activity causes the carbon dioxide level to drop while under the water

2. **Which one of the following describes the basic pathophysiology of drowning?**
   a) Brain swelling due to excessive fluid intake and resultant respiratory arrest
   b) Electrolyte dilution resulting in cardiac arrhythmia and respiratory arrest
   c) Lung injury resulting in hypoxia and possibly cardiac and neurologic injury
   d) Increased compliance and elasticity of the lungs leading to hypoxia
   e) Respiratory difficulty due to pneumonia caused by bacteria in the aspirated water

3. **A 30-year-old male dives headfirst off a cliff into a lake. He surfaces within 5 seconds but is floating and appears to be unconscious. Which one of the following is the most likely etiology for his symptoms?**
   a) He aspirated a large amount of water when he went into the water and became hypoxic
   b) He hyperventilated before jumping in the water and suffered and arrest due to an increased blood carbon dioxide level
   c) He suffered a cardiac arrest due to the suddenness coldness of the water
   d) He suffered a cardiac arrest due to aspiration of hypotonic water and electrolyte dilution
   e) He suffered a cervical injury with resultant paralysis by striking the bottom of the lake

4. **Which one of the following is <u>not</u> part of the management of the drowning victim in the field setting?**
   a) Heimlich maneuver to increase stomach emptying
   b) Immediate CPR if the patient is not breathing
   c) Scene assessment to ensure the area is safe to rescue the victim
   d) Stabilization of the cervical spine if there is concern of injury
   e) Thorough assessment of the respiratory system if the patient is awake

5. **Which one of the following is <u>not</u> a method to help prevent drowning?**
   a) All rafters should wear personal flotation devices
   b) Alcohol should be consumed in moderation when around the water
   c) Camp sites should be established far away from water, especially when children are present
   d) Swimming pools should be surrounded by a 5-foot fence
   e) Those working around or on water should have CPR and water rescue skills

ANSWERS

1. d 2. c 3. E 4. A 5. B

CHAPTER 11

Evacuation Guidelines

This chapter discusses the all-important issue of when to evacuate a sick or injured patient.

Objectives:

- Identify important conditions that might require evacuations
- Recognize signs, symptoms and conditions that require evacuation

Case 1

While on a floating trip on the Warm River in Ashton, Idaho, you come to your drop-off spot to see a group of people surrounding a woman who is in distress. She is lying on the ground and is gasping for air and the breaths she can take make a wheezing sound. You suspect she has eaten a local "wild" berry and perhaps is having a reaction to it. What should you do next?

Case 2

While hiking, you come upon a man who is resting on the side of the trail with a grimace on his face. He claims that his stomach is hurting but he does not know why. What are some questions you should ask him to help you decide when to evacuate him? What findings would alert you to evacuate this person?

BACKGROUND

When to evacuate is one of the biggest and most important decisions in back country medicine

In reality the decision to evacuate a patient is based on a whole variety of factors
- ☐ the length of the evacuation
- ☐ the risk to the patient and to the rescuer
- ☐ the necessity of the evacuation

Some people need to be evacuated for simple injuries such as a foot blister on a hiker

Others are based on the critical nature of the condition, such HACE or HAPE

Others are based on the ability of the patient to be able eat

Some are based on whether or not their condition is likely to become worse

Abdominal Problems

When patients receive serious abdominal injuries, they need to be evacuated immediately.

General evacuation guidelines:
- ☐ Blood appears in the vomit, feces, or urine
- ☐ The pain is associated with the signs and symptoms of shock
- ☐ The pain persists for longer than 24 hours
- ☐ The pain localizes and is there is guarding, rigidity, and tenderness
- ☐ The pain is associated with a fever greater than 102 degrees
- ☐ The pain is associated with pregnancy
- ☐ The patient is unable to drink or eat

Altitude Sickness

Any patient suffering from a lack of control of motor function, HAPE, and/or HACE due to altitude must descend to a lower elevation immediately.

No evacuation is necessary if the patient recovers by descending to a lower elevation.

Allergy Problems

Patients treated for anaphylaxis should be evacuated for further medical evaluation.

Patient should be kept on an oral antihistamine during evacuation.

Animal Bites and Stings

- Patients that are bit or stung by an animal known to be venomous should be evacuated to receive definitive care.
- Large bite wounds, or any wounds suspected of infection, should lead to patient evacuation.

Athletic Injuries

- Evacuation necessity is determined by the patient's ability to use the injured body part. If injury is unusable, the patient should be evacuated, but rapid evacuation is not necessary.

Bleeding

- A patient with signs and symptoms of a rapid decrease in blood pressure, or one who has not quickly improved following treatment of compensatory shock, should be evacuated.
- A patient with irreversible shock should be evacuated as quickly as possible.

Burns

- In the wilderness, the rule of thumb is that a full thickness (third degree) burn that is less than 1% of the TBSA can be treated in the wilderness with proper burn management. This excludes deep burns of the face, hands, feet and genitals. Severe burns greater than 1% should be evacuated.
- In addition, a major burn that meets the following criteria should be evacuated.
  - ☐ Partial thickness (second degree) burns greater than 10% of the TBSA
  - ☐ Full thickness (third degree) burns that are greater than 1% of TBSA
  - ☐ Major burns of the hand, face, feet, or genitals
  - ☐ Burns with inhalation injury
  - ☐ Electric burns
  - ☐ Burns in medically ill patients

Cardiac

- Patients with suspected myocardial infarction and/or congestive heart failure should be evacuated promptly.

Chest Injuries

- Evacuate for any serious chest injury.
- Evacuate promptly if the patient has increasing difficulty breathing and increasing anxiety.

CPR

- Anyone resuscitated by CPR should be evacuated and receive definitive medical care immediately.

Diabetic Emergencies

- Hyperglycemic patients should be evacuated if treatment is not working.
- Hypoglycemic patients should be evaluated for evacuation based on effectiveness of treatment and the patient's wishes.

Dislocations

- Due to the possibility of underlying damage, all dislocations should be evacuated and receive further medical evaluation.
- Promptly evacuate patients who resist reduction attempts.
- Evacuation is not necessary for dislocation of the fingers or for chronic dislocations if the patient still has use of the joint after relocation.

Diving

- Immediate evacuation is required for any patients with decompression sickness or blood clots.
- Sudden unconsciousness or increasing difficulty breathing should lead to prompt evacuation.

Fractures

- Evacuate any patient with suspected fractures.
- Prompt evacuation is necessary with open fractures, fractures of the pelvis or femur, or fractures with decreased motion further from the injury.

Head Injuries

- With a suspected skull fracture or penetrating head wound, patient should be rapidly evacuated.

Heat-Related Problems

- Any patient treated for heat stroke should be evacuated.
- Recovery from heat cramps or heat exhaustion does not necessitate evacuation.

Hypothermia and Frostbite

- A patient recovering from mild or moderate hypothermia does not require evacuation.
- Patients with severe hypothermia should be quickly and carefully evacuated.
- Evacuate any patient with frostbite that results in blisters and/or dusky or blue-gray skin.
- Evacuate if patient has full-thickness frostbite.

Infection

If the patient does not show prompt improvement to treatment of infection, then the patient should be quickly evacuated.

Lightning

Any person involved in a lightning strike should be evacuated, as symptoms might not appear for several days.

Neurologic Emergencies

Evacuate any patient suffering a stroke or minor stroke or who has experienced a seizure.

A significant change in mental status should lead to patient evacuation.

Poisons

Patients with a change of level of consciousness or respiratory drive should be rapidly evacuated.

A known lethal dose of a poison should also lead to immediate evacuation.

Pregnancy

Any possibility of pregnancy complications should lead to patient evacuation.

If a baby is delivered in the wilderness, both the mother and the baby should be evacuated.

Psychiatric

Significant changes in any person's ability to adapt after a crisis or critical incident, violent, suicidal, or psychotic behavior should lead to patient evacuation.

Pulmonary

Patients treated for medical emergencies that involve difficulty breathing should be evacuated immediately.

Patients with mild to moderate asthma or hyperventilation syndrome that is successfully treated do not need to be evacuated.

Shock

A patient with shock, or one who has not quickly improved following treatment of compensatory shock, should be evacuated.

Spine

- A patient with possible spine injury should be evacuated as soon as possible.

Submersion

- Patients involved in accidental submersion, especially if they lost consciousness, required resuscitation, have difficulty breathing, or have a history of lung disease, need to receive further evaluation in a medical setting.
- Immediate evacuation is necessary for a patient who remains unconscious following a submersion incident.

Wounds

- Evacuation should be prompt when there is a high probability of infection or deep wounds.
- Shock from blood loss that is not reversed by treatment should be quickly evacuated.

QUESTIONS

1. While on a campout, a friend of yours falls into the campfire and sustains a burn on his right hand. The burn appears to be deep enough to be considered a third degree burn but occurred only on his right palm and the palmar surface of his fifth finger (pinky), which you estimate to be less than 1% of his TBSA. What is the recommendation for evacuation in this situation?
   a) He can be treated with a wilderness medicine burn kit because his burn occurred over less than 1% of his body area.
   b) He should be evacuated and taken to a hospital for treatment.
   c) With rest, water, and some Neosporin he should be fine.
   d) Wrap the wound for now and if it becomes worse within the next 24-48 hrs, evacuate.

2. Which of the following is NOT a situation where a patient needs to be evacuated due to an abdominal injury?
   a) The pain persists for longer than 24 hours
   b) The pain localizes and is there is guarding, rigidity, and tenderness
   c) Blood appears in the vomit, feces or urine
   d) The patient has watery diarrhea

3. You are on a backpacking trip in the Uintas when a man in your group faints and falls to the ground. You and a friend perform the ABC's and perform CPR. He is resuscitated after the first attempt. He did not sustain any injuries from falling to the ground and states afterward that he feels okay to continue with the hike; he just needs to rest a few hours. What is the proper course of action in this case?
   a) Evacuate him immediately and seek medical attention.
   b) Evacuate him immediately, and have him stay home resting or close to a hospital for 24 hours.
   c) Have him rest for four hours, then continue the hike but at a much slower pace.
   d) Continue the hike, but at a much slower pace.

4. While biking in Moab, a friend falls from his bike and dislocates his shoulder. One of the people in your group is a physical therapist and relocates his shoulder. After the successful relocation, your friend is able to move his shoulder. Your friend says that this happens to him all the time. What should be done next?
   a) Evacuate him immediately and seek medical attention.
   b) If he does not have further problems with his shoulder, he does not need to be evacuated.
   c) Do not let him ride anymore. Finish your riding and if possible, evacuate your friend.
   d) Attempt to re-dislocate his shoulder and reset it several times. This should help prevent future dislocations.

5. **You are on a day hike when a friend of yours forgot to bring enough water. After a few hours, he begins to act confused and complains of dizziness and fatigue. You give him some of your water and he is still a bit dizzy, but he does not appear to be confused anymore, just a bit fatigued. What should be done next?**
   a) Let him keep your water bottle and finish up your hike.
   b) You should rest for a few hours to allow him to drink, then continue your hike.
   c) Evacuate him immediately.
   d) Have him run up the trail for a bit to reset his fluid levels and wake himself up.

ANSWERS
1. b 2. d 3. a 4. b 5. C

CHAPTER 12

Eye Injuries and Disorders

This chapter will train you to recognize and treat eye injuries and disorders according to the following criteria:

- How to best treat injuries to tissues surrounding the eye, including those that are worrisome for a more significant injury
- To recognize ocular injuries and to understand their basic management in the wilderness
- To describe evaluation and treatment of the patient with a red eye
- To understand the possible diagnoses associated with visual loss
- To describe evacuation criteria for the patient with an eye injury or complaint

Case 1

A 29-year-old male is fishing with friends at a river three hours away from the nearest hospital. The hike from the car is 10 minutes on a flat trail. After a cast, the man falls down, writhing in pain. His friends notice that the fishing line is attached to the hook, which has punctured the victim's eye. He has difficulty holding still and cannot open the eye because of pain and anxiety.

1. What is the next step in managing this patient?
2. What do you do with the fishing hook?
3. Can this be dealt with in the wilderness?
4. If evacuation is necessary, what is the best way to proceed?

Case 2

A 59-year-old male complains of a sudden decrease in vision in his left eye. He was fine several minutes previously, but then he saw flashing lights in the left eye, followed by "floaters." He is able to see, but his vision seems decreased. On examination, his eye appears to be completely normal and he is easily able to count fingers at six feet in front of him.

1. What is the next step in managing this patient?
2. Can you manage him in the wilderness or does he need to be evacuated?
3. If evacuation is necessary, should you place a shield over his eye?

Case 3

A 32-year-old woman is struck in the right eye by a rock while climbing up a cliff. Other than a small contusion on her eyelid, there is no external trauma. Examination of her eye shows normal counting of fingers at six feet and a very small layer of blood overlying the iris along the lower border of the cornea. The remainder of the exam is normal.

1. What is the injury?
2. What are the potential complications from this injury?
3. Is it reasonable to give the victim ibuprofen for pain?
4. Can you manage the victim in the wilderness, or does she need to be evacuated?
5. If evacuation is necessary, should you place a shield over her eye?

PERIOCULAR TRAUMA

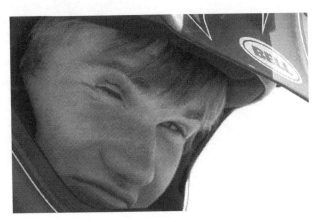

Figure 12.1 Superficial Lid Laceration

Superficial lid laceration

- A superficial lid laceration does not penetrate the full thickness of the eyelid and does not include the lid margins or the eye itself.
- Penetration of the eye by a foreign object must be ruled out.
- Treatment of superficial lid lacerations is the same as that for other minor lacerations.
  - ☐ Use clean gauze to apply pressure to the cut to stop the bleeding. However, it is important not to put pressure on the eye but rather on the surrounding bones of the orbit.
  - ☐ After the bleeding stops, strongly irrigate the wound with clean water or saline solution to remove dirt or foreign objects.
  - ☐ Apply bacitracin ointment in a thin ribbon to the wound and attempt to close the laceration with tape strips. Cover the wound with a sterile non-adherent dressing or gauze and tape the dressing in place.
  - ☐ Monitor daily for signs of infection, such as redness, swelling, pain, and pus. Depending on the severity of the laceration, evacuation may be necessary for definitive repair.

Complex lid laceration

- A complex lid laceration penetrates the full thickness of the lid and/or includes the lid margins.
- Penetration of the globe must be ruled out.
- Use sterile gauze to stop the bleeding. Irrigate the cut with saline solution or clean water if saline is not available. Saline is preferable, since irrigating a complex lid laceration will most likely include irrigating the eye.
- Most health care providers are not comfortable closing complex lid lacerations. There is a considerable risk of poor outcome if the laceration is not closed appropriately. In cases where the treating health care provider is not qualified or confident about closing the wound, the wound should be treated with antibiotic ointment and then kept covered.
- Due to the need for repair, patients with complex lid lacerations should be evacuated if possible.

Blunt trauma

Blunt force to the globe or surrounding bony orbit and soft tissues can fracture the thin bones that hold the eye in place.

In most cases, significant periocular bruising and swelling will occur.

There may also be restriction of eye movements, which is called *entrapment*.

Significant swelling, restricted eye movements, clear fluid leaking from of the nose, and decreased vision following blunt trauma to the orbit suggest considerable damage. The victim should be evacuated for evaluation and treatment.

OCULAR TRAUMA

Penetrating foreign body

If a foreign object has penetrated the eye, do not try to remove it. Stabilize the object by taping a sterile dressing in a donut shape around the eye and then taping a cup or pair of glasses over the eye to prevent any jarring of the embedded object.

You may consider patching the other eye shut to prevent eye movement if the victim does not have to use his or her sight to navigate out of the wilderness. However, in most cases this is unpractical.

If the eye has been punctured, resulting in an open globe, and no foreign object is present, a protective shield should be taped over the eye. Sunglasses can function as a shield by being taped over both eyes.

In any possible case of globe penetration, it is important not to put any pressure on the damaged eye. External pressure may raise intraocular pressure, resulting in expulsion of intraocular structures. An open globe injury is a true emergency and should result in immediate evacuation to prevent infection and vision loss.

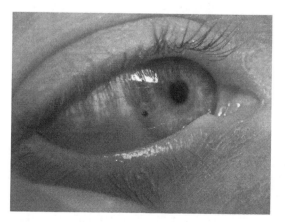

Figure 12.2 Penetrating Foreign Body

Corneal abrasion

This is a disruption of the epithelial layer of the cornea.

It is most commonly caused by trauma, although it may occur "spontaneously" in individuals who have had a recently healed abrasion.

A corneal abrasion may result in moderate to severe pain, tearing, and sensitivity to light.

Treatment:

- Evaluate the eye to ensure there is not a globe perforation or retained foreign body on the cornea.
- Apply a topical ophthalmic antibiotic ointment or liquid if such is available. If an antibiotic is not available, the abrasion should still heal well.
- Consider patching the eye for comfort.
  - This is done by tightly taping a piece of gauze from the forehead to the cheekbone.
  - Eye patching is not a necessity, but some victims report that this gives provides relief from their symptoms. Others may find that the eye patch is irritating and request to remain without the patch, which is fine.

The epithelial layer of the cornea heals rapidly, usually within 24 to 72 hours.

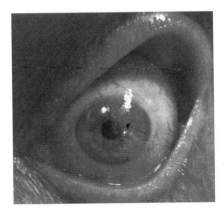

Figure 12.3 Corneal abrasion

Ultraviolet radiation burns (Sunburn of the eye)

The protective layer of the cornea is easily damaged by exposure to ultraviolet radiation from direct sunlight, reflection off snow, or reflection off water.

Symptoms are mild to severe eye pain, reddened eyes, sensitivity to light, tearing, blurry vision, and foreign body sensation in the eye 6 to 10 hours after exposure.

These symptoms commonly involve both eyes, which is a clue to this diagnosis.

This injury is easily prevented with sunglasses with side shields. Always wear proper eye protection in bright light, especially when light is reflected off snow or water.

Non-penetrating foreign body

Non-penetrating foreign bodies can result in pain and irritation. If natural tearing does not clear the eye of the foreign body, irrigating the eye with saline solution is sometimes successful. Larger chunks can be removed from the conjunctiva with a cotton swab.

Do not attempt to remove foreign objects embedded in the eye. If an object persists ior cannot be removed from the conjunctiva, apply a strip of bacitracin ointment to the lower lid. If necessary for pain control, patch the eye as for a corneal abrasion. If there is any suggestion of an infection, do not patch the eye. Evacuation will be necessary because corneal foreign bodies can cause permanent scarring and conjunctival foreign bodies can become infected.

Hyphema (blood in front of the lens)

■ A hyphema is a collection of blood in the anterior chamber of the eye that is in front of the lens The anterior chamber is the fluid-filled space between the cornea and iris. A larger hyphema may be noted by visualizing a layer of blood overlying the iris along the bottom margin of the iris.

■ Hyphema is a serious condition that mandates evacuation due to its potential complications, which include acute glaucoma and rebleeding. Use an eye shield to protect the eye from any further trauma. Avoid aspirin, ibuprofen, or any other medications that may cause more bleeding. Activity should also be restricted as much as possible during evacuation.

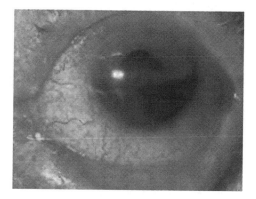

Figure 12.4 Hyphema

ACUTE VISION LOSS IN A NORMAL APPEARING EYE

■ It is possible for a victim to lose vision in an eye that looks completely normal. There are various causes of acute vision loss. Each is serious and can result in permanent vision loss. Whenever visual acuity dramatically decreases, or there is a sudden loss of vision, evacuate the victim immediately.

Retinal detachment

■ Retinal detachment occurs when the retina (the innermost, posterior layer of the eye) detaches from the middle layer) This may be because of trauma or may occur spontaneously. It is more common in people with severe nearsightedness because of the shape of their eyes.

■ Initial symptoms commonly include a sensation of flashing lights followed by a shower of "floaters." Over time, this may lead to a shadow in any part of the visual field. Left untreated, this can spread to involve the entire visual field within a short period of time. Surgical intervention can help to preserve vision, so prompt evacuation must ensue shortly after initial symptoms are noted.

ACUTE RED EYE

Subconjunctival hemorrhage

- Subconjunctival hemorrhage is accumulation of blood in the space between the conjunctiva and sclera.
- This results in an extremely red-looking ("bloodshot") eye but is rarely a serious condition.
- This condition may occur spontaneously or as a result of increased intrathoracic pressure, such as that which occurs with straining or coughing.
- It normally resolves over a period of a few days to two weeks without treatment.
- If this occurs from trauma, examine the eye for other more serious conditions, such as a foreign body or puncture.

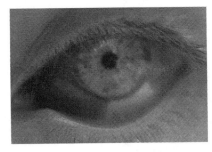 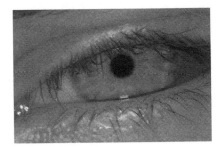

Figure 12.5 Subconjunctival Hemorrhage

Conjunctivitis (Infection on the surface of the eye)

- The major causes of conjunctivitis are viral, bacterial, and allergic.
- Acute bacterial conjunctivitis is much less common than is viral conjunctivitis.
- Viral and allergic conjunctivitis usually require no treatment. In the wilderness, the most practical treatment for the symptoms of these conditions is cold compresses if ice or a cool wet cloth is available.
- Bacterial conjunctivitis is most often treated with a broad-spectrum ophthalmic ointment or suspension.
- Since the cause of conjunctivitis may be difficult to diagnose, if inflammation becomes worse after a few days, it may be appropriate to evacuate for evaluation and treatment.
- If a red eye is accompanied by decreased visual acuity or if the cornea becomes opaque or cloudy, evacuation is necessary because these latter symptoms possibly denote more serious ocular disease.

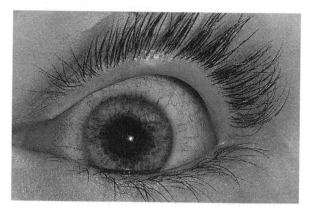

Figure 12.6 Conjunctivitis

EVACUATION GUIDELINES

- Evacuate immediately if the globe has been perforated.
- Evacuate immediately if there is a sudden loss of vision in a normal-appearing eye.
- Evacuate as soon as possible if there is a complex lid laceration or hyphema, or if the cornea becomes cloudy.

QUESTIONS

1. You are on a camping trip when a 60-year-old male awakens in the morning up with a red eye. He does not complain of vision loss and in fact does not notice any problem until you bring it to his attention. What is the next best step?
   a) Apply direct pressure to the eye
   b) Evacuate immediately
   c) Monitor for signs of vision loss or pain
   d) Apply ointment and patch the eye
   e) Irrigate the eye with saline or clean water

2. On a youth wilderness excursion, a young man is struck in the forehead with a tree branch during a robust game of tag. The victim falls on the ground and complains of severe eye pain. A small dry twig is lodged in the white part of the eye and does not fall out. Before evacuating, what should be done?
   a) Apply direct pressure to the eye
   b) Give the patient aspirin
   c) Remove the twig and patch the eye
   d) Apply ointment and patch the eye
   e) Do not remove the twig and tape a shield over the eye

3. The morning after a long day of river rafting, a 58-year-old female complains of having seen light flashes during the night even with her eyes closed. Now, in the daytime, with her eyes open she sees dark dirt-like spots in one field of vision. What is the next best step?
   a) Apply direct pressure to the eye
   b) Evacuate immediately
   c) Monitor over time for signs of vision loss
   d) Apply ointment and patch the eye
   e) Irrigate the eye with saline or clean water

4. It is beginning to become dark on a trail and you accidentally walk into a low-lying branch that scrapes your eye. You feel intense pain that makes it difficult to open your eye. During the brief moments when you eye is open, you notice your vision to be unchanged. What is the next best step?
   a) Apply direct pressure to the eye
   b) Apply ointment, patch the eye, and evacuate immediately
   c) Apply ointment, patch the eye, and reassess in the morning
   d) Take acetaminophen for pain control and keep hiking
   e) Rinse the eye with clean river water, apply ointment, patch the eye, and reassess in the morning

5. **A young man slips while rock climbing. During the fall, he scrapes his face on a sharp rock and is cut on his right upper eyelid below the brow. The cut is bleeding profusely, but his eye movements are normal and the only pain is felt on the surface. What is the best treatment?**
   a) Apply direct pressure to the cut, with pressure over the bone, and treat like a normal skin laceration
   b) Apply direct pressure to the cut, with pressure over the eye, and treat like a normal skin laceration
   c) Give aspirin for pain control and evacuate

ANSWERS 1. e 2. e 3. b 4. e 5. a

CHAPTER 13

Gender-Specific Emergencies

Objectives:

- Learn the common genitourinary conditions that affect males and females in the wilderness.
- Understand the basic treatments of these conditions.
- Learn when patients need to be evacuated.

Case

While backpacking on a three-day hike, you notice one of your friends begins to have abdominal pains. She says she hasn't had these before and they seem quite painful. During your secondary assessment you question her about recent illnesses and she tells you that she is four months pregnant but didn't want to tell anyone because she has already had two miscarriages. What should you do? What are some other gender-specific emergencies like this that you should be aware of in the backcountry?

Introduction

Pelvic pain or Injuries to the genitalia can be embarrassing, frightening, and even life threatening. When talking to a patient, you should find a private place to talk. Also, avoid using technical terminology and slang, and always have a member of the patient's sex present during any exams.

MALE SPECIFIC EMERGENCIES

Male Anatomy

- **Penis and scrotum** – visible external genitalia
- **Urethra** – expels urine and semen
- **Testes** – site of sperm and testosterone production
- **Epididymis** – runs behind testes, carries sperm
- **Ductus deferens** – carries sperm from epididymis to ejaculatory duct

Inguinal Hernia

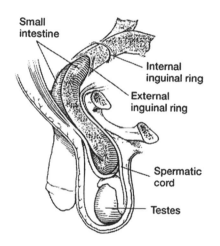

*Figure 13.1 Inguinal Hernia with Intestines
Protruding Into Scrotum*

Inguinal hernia occurs when part of the intestine pushes into the scrotum or groin.

An inguinal hernia can be caused by birth defects, aging, or trauma, as well as increased abdominal pressure.

Swelling and or lumping in the groin/scrotum along with sharp and steady pain are indications of an inguinal hernia.

If a patient has an inguinal hernia, attempt to reduce hernia with moderate, steady, upward pressure for 10+ minutes.

Complications

- ☐ Incarceration- unable to reduce bowel
- ☐ Strangulation- blood supply to bowel interrupted causing ischemia.

☐ Intestinal Blockage- prevents the normal passage of intestinal contents

■ **When to evacuate** – unable to put hernia back in place, reappears, evidence of any complications listed above then evacuate the patient.

Epididymitis

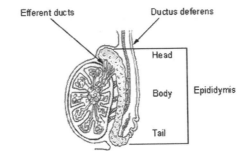

Sagittal section of a testis and Epididymis

Figure 13.2 Anatomy of the Testicle

☐ Epididymitis is the swelling of the epididymis.

☐ Epididymitis is caused by gonorrhea, syphilis, tuberculosis, mumps, or prostatitis. Epididymitis is not caused by trauma.

☐ Symptoms include fever, pain in the scrotum, and redness and swelling.

☐ The best treatment for epididymitis is bed rest, support of the scrotum (jock strap), ibuprofen, and antibiotics. Therefore, evacuation is necessary.

Torsion of the Testis

☐ Torsion of the testis refers to the twisting of the testicles and the associated blood vessels within the scrotum. This cuts off the blood supply to the testis.

☐ Torsion of the testis occurs from various movements that can jostle the testis.

☐ A sign that a patient has torsion of the testis is sudden severe pain to the point where any movement may be unbearable. Also, the scrotum may be red and swollen and the testis may be elevated on the affected side.

☐ If torsion of the testis has occurred, immediate evacuation is necessary to untwist the blood vessels and restore blood flow. Evacuation may be made more difficult due to the patient's inability to walk. Cool compresses may help to alleviate the pain to a more manageable level.

☐ If the patient is unable to walk and there is delayed evacuation of more than two to three hours, on-site treatment may be necessary. In this case, attempt to rotate testicle back into position (typically requires an "outward" rotation).

☐ If this doesn't work, rotate the testicles two turns in the opposite direction.

☐ Note that the patient may want to do these treatments himself.

FEMALE SPECIFIC EMERGENCIES

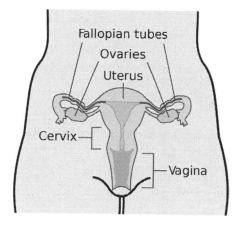

Figure 13.3 Anatomy of the Pelvis

Female Anatomy

Female reproductive organs lie within the pelvic cavity

- **Vagina** – three to four inch birth canal; continuously moistened (clean, acidic)
- **Cervix** – top of the vagina with a small hole leading to the uterus
- **Uterus** – size of fist, located between bladder and rectum
- **Ovaries** – located four to five inches below waist; produces eggs, estrogen, and progesterone
- **Fallopian tubes** – carries egg to uterus
- **Fimbria** – finger-like projections at the end of the fallopian tubes; sweep egg from ovary into tubes

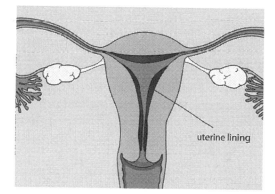

Figure 13.4 Anatomy of the Uterus and Ovaries

The Menstrual Cycle
The menstrual cycle is the monthly release of ova that typically starts at 12 years of age lasting until menopause around age 50. Along with the release of ova there are also four to six tablespoons of blood, tissue, and mucus that are expelled from the body.

Phases of the Menstrual Cycle:
☐ **Days 1-5:** Endometrial tissue sloughs off the uterus and is expelled through the vagina – this is commonly referred to as the "period."

☐ **Days 6-16:** Endometrial tissue regrows with ovulation on day 14. During this time there is a rich blood supply to the uterus.

☐ **Days 17-28:** Estrogen and progesterone levels fall (assuming no pregnancy exists) and the lining of uterus begins to shed, which leads to a decline in blood supply to the uterus.

Mittelschmerz

Mittelschmerz is the term given to the pain that occurs during the middle part of the menstrual cycle due to ovulation.

Symptoms include sudden, sharp, moderate to severe pain on the left or right side of the lower abdomen. The location of the pain imitates the pain experienced during acute appendicitis.

Treatment of mittelschmerz includes over-the-counter pain medications and general emotional support, as well as monitoring for signs of other problems.

Dysmenorrhea

This is the term assigned to pain during menstruation.

Dysmenorrhea can be caused by prostaglandins, endometriosis, pelvic inflammatory disease (PID), or anatomic abnormalities.

Cramping, general discomfort, and pain are typical symptoms of dysmenorrhea.

Ibuprofen, relaxation techniques, massage, heat, and exercise are all acceptable treatments.

Secondary Amenorrhea

Secondary amenorrhea is the absence of a menstrual period after a woman has had at least one period, which can be caused by pregnancy, ovarian tumors, intense athletic training, altitude, and/or stress.

Please take note that changes in menstrual cycles are common on wilderness expeditions and may just be normal adjustments to a new activity.

Premenstrual Syndrome (PMS)

Premenstrual syndrome is the cluster of symptoms occurring just prior to menstruation.

The specific cause of premenstrual syndrome is unknown but has been described as a physiological mechanism.

Signs and symptoms of PMS include depression, anxiety, breast tenderness, food cravings, headache, fatigue, bloating, and edema.

Over-the-counter pain medications, diet modifications, decreased stress level, Vitamin B6, and exercise all help to treat PMS.

Vaginal Infections

Vaginal infections include yeast, bacterial, or trichomonal infection of the vagina which can be caused by lowered body resistance, a diet high in sugar, antibiotics, diabetics, cuts and abrasions, sexually transmitted infections, and inadequate hygiene.

Symptoms of a vaginal infection are excessive or malodorous discharge from the vagina, redness, soreness, itching, and burning on urination.

In some cases of vaginal infections there is the need to restore the appropriate level of acidity of the vagina, which can be accomplished with a douche. Over-the-counter medications such as Monistat are also effective for some types of infection.

☐ Please note that women with trichomonas or other sexually transmitted infections may require antibiotic treatment. A physician should ultimately treat ongoing infections after evacuation.

Other treatments of vaginal infections include Acetaminophen and warm or cool compresses.

Evacuate if no improvement occurs in 48 hours.

There are measures that can be taken to prevent vaginal infections:

☐ Clean perineal area with soap and water daily.
☐ Wear cotton underwear and loose pants.
☐ Avoid coffee, alcohol, and sugar.

Urinary Tract Infections

Urinary tract infections are very common in women.

The symptoms include increased frequency/urgency of urination with little urine output, burning on urination, and pain above pubic bone.

The best treatments for urinary tract infections are antibiotics, drinking lots of water, frequent urination, and cleaning with water and mild soap. Eating cranberries, prunes, and plums can also help.

Evacuate the patient if the infection lasts for more than 48 hours.

Pelvic Inflammatory Disease (PID)

PID is an inflammation of the fallopian tubes, peritoneum, ovaries, and/or uterus and is caused by gonorrhea, chlamydia, and/or enteric bacteria.

Common symptoms that accompany PID that will help to diagnose are diffuse pain in middle of lower abdomen, fever, nausea, vomiting, vaginal discharge, irregular bleeding, and pain/bleeding during intercourse.

If you encounter a case of pelvic inflammatory disease in the wilderness, you should evacuate immediately and seek further medical care.

Toxic Shock Syndrome (TSS)

TSS is the result of a bacterial infection that occurs when a tampon is left in place for a prolonged period of time. The bacteria most commonly responsible, *staph. aureus*, release an inflammatory toxin into the patient's body.

Signs and symptoms of TSS include abrupt onset of high fever, abdominal pain, sore throat, nausea and vomiting, and muscle aches. A very evident symptom of toxic shock syndrome is a sunburn-like rash over most of the body with the mucus membranes a deep beet red color.

The treatment for TSS is to remove the tampon immediately. Also, drink lots of liquids and evacuate immediately to seek further medical attention.

The best treatment of TSS is prevention!

OBSTETRICAL EMERGENCIES

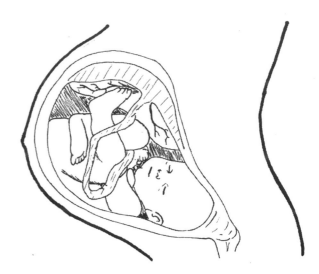

- The best way to avoid obstetrical emergencies in the wilderness/backcountry is to advise pregnant women to avoid traveling in the wilderness during the last four to six weeks of pregnancy.
- Normal Pregnancy lasts about 40 weeks.
- The signs and symptoms of pregnancy are:
  - ☐ Absence of anticipated menstrual period
  - ☐ Unusual fatigue
  - ☐ Morning sickness – nausea and vomiting
  - ☐ Breast tenderness and enlargement
  - ☐ Frequent Urination

Premature Labor

- Definition is birth at 37 weeks or less of gestation
- The causes are unclear
- Most delivers in the wilderness will be premature since women near the end of pregnancy do not travel typically
- Lungs are not fully developed, they are unable to stay warm and their might be more blood loss in the mother
- Premature infants are more fragile then term infants

How to Deliver a Baby

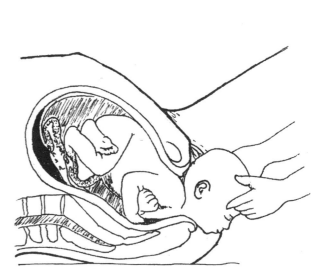

- Always ask how many children has the mother had. The more children, the faster the process becomes.
- A good position is with the mother on her hands and knees or with the mother in the lateral recumbent position.
- Three stages of labor:
  - ☐ Stage 1: this lasts about 8 – 12 hours where the cervix will efface and dilate.
  - ☐ Stage 2: this lasts from 30 minutes to about 2 hours. The baby will move through and deliver through the birth canal.
  - ☐ State 3: 5 – 10 minutes after the baby is delivered, the placenta will be delivered.
- Clean your hands and mothers perineal area with soap and water
- Look into the birth canal and see if you can see the baby's head – if the feet are coming first this becomes a huge problem and immediate evacuation is essential
- You might have to help part the vaginal tissue to help avoid tearing
- At this point encourage the mother to push between contractions, not at their peak
- Support the baby's head – do not pull it as nerve damage can result
- The baby's head will rotate on it own, once this is done, the baby will emerge quick as the shoulders have moved through the birth canal

- [ ] Reddish water will gush out at this point.
- [ ] If cord is wrapped around neck, unwrap it immediately
- [ ] Place baby on mother's chest
- [ ] Tie with string or rope in two places and cut in between
- [ ] Several minutes after infant the placenta will separate from the uterine wall
- [ ] Apply gentle contraction on the umbilical cord until placenta is delivered
- [ ] You can massage the abdomen/uterus to minimize bleeding
- [ ] 98% of all babies are delivered without complications
- [ ] After delivery evacuation is immediate

QUESTIONS

1. **Which of the following accurately describes toxic shock syndrome?**
   a) A reaction to eating processed food that causes stomach discomfort and sweating
   b) An infection by the bacteria *staph. aureus* that gives the patient a sunburn-like rash and red mucous membranes
   c) A low blood volume state probably due to ingesting wild berries
   d) A state of delirium and agitation after years of eating non-organic foods

2. **If a person is in a situation where they are unable to get a course of antibiotics to treat a urinary tract infection (e.g., days away from civilization), what is a good treatment?**
   a) Drink lots of water, clean the area, and perhaps consume sources of cranberries, prunes, and plums
   b) Consuming acidic fruits such as oranges and tomatoes to lower the urine pH and kill the bacteria
   c) Placing a cloth boiled in hot water in the infected area, which should pull the infected bacteria in by osmosis
   d) Ingesting mold which may overgrow the area too but it will out-compete the bacteria

3. **What is pelvic inflammatory disease?**
   a) An inflammatory condition of the superior crest of the iliac bone
   b) Inflammation of the urinary tract
   c) Inflammation of fallopian tubes, peritoneum, ovaries, and/or uterus
   d) Inflammation of the nerves supplying pelvic structures

4. **What are the symptoms of pelvic inflammatory disease?**
   a) Diffuse pain in middle of lower abdomen, fever, nausea and vomiting, irregular bleeding, and pain/bleeding during intercourse
   b) Headache, shooting pain into the lower abdomen, and abdominal flushing
   c) Stabbing pain in the lower abdomen, pain with exercise and exertion, and dizziness
   d) Burning in the lower abdomen, fatigue, malaise, and lower extremity cramping

5. **A young lady becomes anxious and consumes more food than usual for a two-day period. She develops a headache and feels like she doesn't want to do anything she usually does. A day later she menstruates and her symptoms subside. What does this vignette describe?**
   a) Pelvic inflammatory disease
   b) Premenstrual syndrome
   c) Urinary tract infection
   d) Toxic shock syndrome

ANSWERS
1. b 2. a 3. c 4. a 5. b

CHAPTER 14

Head Trauma and Spine Injuries

Objectives:

- Know basic brain anatomy
- Be able to recognize common head injuries
- Be able to treat common head injuries
- Know basic spine anatomy
- Know common mechanisms of how the spinal cord is injured
- Know initial treatment for spinal cord injures

Case

During a hike a 20-year-old female falls off of a small boulder and hits her head. She loses consciousness for a brief moment. She awakes and is bleeding from the side of her head. She had scarped her back.

1. What is the initial management of this patient?
2. What are the major concerns to watch for?
3. How do you treat the head wound?

HEAD TRAUMA

Brain Anatomy

- Cerebrum – center of higher function
- Cerebellum – equilibrium and coordination
- Brain Stem – vital metabolic functions
- Meninges – membranes covering the brain & spinal cord
  - ☐ Dura Mater
  - ☐ Arachnoid Mater
  - ☐ Pia Mater
- Cerebrospinal fluid – provides a cushion for the brain and spinal cord, It circulates under the arachnoid mater called the subarachnoid space

Scalp Laceration

- Scalp lacerations are common and when they occur they typically will bleed profusely.
- This is very concerning to those around the victim.
  - ☐ The bleeding is because of the blood-rich nature of the scalp.
  - ☐ Scalp blood vessels typically do not constrict rapidly to slow bleeding, as is the case in other areas of the skin.
- The best was to stop the bleeding is with direct pressure from a bulky dressing.
  - ☐ Bulky dressing will disperse pressure to help prevent pressing bone fragments into the brain
- Clean the wound thoroughly with water when possible.
- Clip hair if needed to visualize wound if needed.
  - ☐ However, do not shave the hair, as this may increase the risk of infection
- Closure
  - ☐ Butterfly bandages or skin closure strips work well.
  - ☐ Apply the strips perpendicular to wound.
  - ☐ Pull wound together, but not too tight.
  - ☐ Dress with antibiotic ointment and sterile gauze
  - ☐ Monitor for signs and symptoms of infection

Concussions

- Patients with mild head injuries typically have concussions.
- A concussion is defined as physiologic injury to the brain without any evidence of structural alteration.
- Typical symptoms include:
  - ☐ Confusion
  - ☐ Amnesia
  - ☐ Vertigo
  - ☐ Nausea/vomiting
  - ☐ Disorientation
  - ☐ Slurred speech
  - ☐ Loss of consciousness

☐ Very emotional
☐ Headache

If a concussion is suspected then those displaying persistent vomiting, severe headache, amnesia of loss of consciousness should be evacuated

Skull Fracture

Skull fractures may occur with head injuries.

While the skull is tough and provides excellent protection for the brain, a severe impact or blow can result in fracture of the skull.

It may be accompanied by injury to the brain.

The brain can be affected directly by damage to the nervous system tissue and bleeding. The brain can also be affected indirectly by blood clots that form under the skull and then compress the underlying brain tissue (subdural or epidural hematoma).

A simple fracture is a break in the bone without damage to the skin.

A linear skull fracture is a break in a cranial bone resembling a thin line, without splintering, depression, or distortion of bone.

A depressed skull fracture is a break in a cranial bone (or "crushed" portion of skull) with depression of the bone in toward the brain.

Signs and symptoms

Decreased level of consciousness
Fracture lines visible beneath a tear in the scalp
Deformity (often a depression) at the injury site
Possible "Raccoon eyes" (black and blue discoloration around eyes)
Possible Battle's sign (black and blue discoloration behind and below the ears)
Seizures
CSF leaking from nose or ears

Treatment

Do not attempt to stop the flow of fluid from nose/ears
This may be the body's way of decreasing ICP
Impaled objects should NOT be removed
Bleeding should be allowed to continue to help allow decrease brain pressure
DON'T apply direct pressure
Stabilize object in place with large bulky dressings
Patient should be evacuated immediately

Closed Head Injury

This is from a violent impact to head that does not fracture the skull
Such trauma often involves a period of unconsciousness
It almost always involves damage to brain cells
The severity of the injury depends on:

- ☐ The duration of the unconsciousness
- ☐ The depth of the unconsciousness
- Bleeding inside the head results in increased intracranial pressure (ICP) that can result in permanent brain damage or death
- Contusion (bruise) to the brain can lead to swelling, which can increase ICP
- Epidural hematoma – this is bleeding above the dura
  - ☐ This is almost arterial thus has a high pressure then venous bleeding
  - ☐ This usually causes a rapid rise in ICP and quick death
- Subdural hematoma – this is bleeding below the dura
  - ☐ This is usually venous bleeding and at lower pressure
  - ☐ Causes a slow rise in ICP and can lead to death hours or days after the accident
- Increased ICP typically causes:
  - ☐ Mental status changes – disorientation, irritability, combativeness and coma
  - ☐ Heart rate slows
- Respiratory rate
  - ☐ Early: erratic changes
  - ☐ Late: rapid and deep breathing
  - ☐ Increased blood pressure
  - ☐ Flushed skin
  - ☐ Headache
  - ☐ Visual disturbances
  - ☐ Excessive sleepiness
  - ☐ Protracted nausea and vomiting
  - ☐ Ataxia (loss of balance)
  - ☐ Seizures
  - ☐ Unequal pupils
  - ☐ Rigid body postures

Treatment of Head Injuries

- No loss of consciousness
  - ☐ Mostly stable with rare chance of serious problems
  - ☐ Monitor patient for 24 hours especially if there was a loss of consciousness
  - ☐ Evacuate if signs of serious brain damage develop
- Momentary loss of consciousness
  - ☐ Monitor closely for 24 hours - patient has sustained some brain cell damage.
  - ☐ Wake patient every couple of hours to monitor
  - ☐ Evacuate if signs of serious brain damage develop
- Long-term loss of consciousness
  - ☐ Evacuate immediately
- When to evacuate may be a difficult decision
  - ☐ If you evacuate anybody knocked unconscious, you will be acting responsibly
  - ☐ If the patient only a momentary loss of consciousness and responds immediately to verbal stimuli and has no signs of brain injury they are probably okay to stay in the wilderness
- Do not give painkilling medications
  - ☐ They may mask the signs and symptoms of a serious brain injury and make it difficulty to diagnosis
  - ☐ Aspirin/NSAIDs may increase bleeding in the brain so avoid these medicines

If you have to leave the patient alone for any reason
- ☐ Ensure that the patient doesn't lose their airway
- ☐ Roll patient on his/her side

SPINE INJURIES

- Spinal cord trauma is damage to the spinal cord.
- It may result from direct injury to the cord itself or indirectly from disease of the surrounding bones, tissues, or blood vessel.

Anatomy of the Spinal Cord and the Spine

- Cervical vertebrae – there are 7 of them – these are numbered from the top C1 – C7
  - ☐ These are the east protected of all the vertebrae
  - ☐ Hence they are the most prone to serious injury
- Thoracic vertebrae – there are 12 of them – these are numbered from the top T1 – T12
  - ☐ These are attached to ribs protecting the organs of the chest
  - ☐ These are protected by the back muscles
- Lumbar vertebrae – there are 5 of them – these are numbered from the top L1 – L5
  - ☐ There are the strongest of the vertebrae but the muscles are prone to injury from lifting and twisting
- Sacral vertebrae
  - ☐ Fused and attached to pelvic girdle
- Coccyx – the bottom part of the sacrum
- The spinal cord passes through vertebral foramen in the middle of each vertebrae
- There are discs of cartilage between each vertebrae allow movement and help absorb shock. In time these tend to degenerate
- Nerve roots branch out from between the vertebrae and send peripheral nerves to the rest of the body

Mechanism of Spine Injuries

- Excessive flexion – diver hits the bottom of a shallow pond
- Excessive extension – whiplash in car accident
- Compression – climber falls and lands sitting
- Distraction – hanging
- Excessive rotation – ski injury
- Excessive lateral bending – stationary skier hit from the side by a high-speed skier
- Penetration injury – stabbing or goring
- Violent deceleration – 30 foot un-roped fall
- Vertebral fractures
- Herniated intervertebral discs
- Swelling of the cord

Assessment of Spinal Injuries

- Treat all unconscious trauma patients as if they have a spinal injury until proven otherwise.
- Initial assessment – is the patient breathing?
  - ☐ If a patient has a spinal cord injury above C4 – they will likely not be breathing!
  - ☐ Patients with spinal cord injuries between C4 and T1 may result in "belly breathing"
- Vital Signs – is the patient in neurogenic shock?
  - ☐ Loss of control over the dilation and constriction of blood vessels due to nerve damage.
  - ☐ Vasoconstricted (cool and pale) above the site of injury
  - ☐ Vasodilated (warm and flushed) below the site of injury

Spinal Cord Injury – Signs and Symptoms

- Most often a spinal cord injury will involve trauma to the cord rather then cutting the cord.
- The symptoms vary from patient to patient and also depend upon the mechanism of injury (MOI)
- A person who falls from a 30-foot cliff is more likely to have significant trauma then someone who slips off a chair.
- If any trauma to the cord is suspected either from the MOI or from the examination, be aggressive in the management of the patient.
- There are some typical signs:
  - ☐ Labored breathing
  - ☐ Signs and symptoms of shock
  - ☐ Altered sensations
    - -Numbness or tingling
    - -Hot or cold sensations
      - § Weakness or paralysis
      - § Pain and/or tenderness along the spine
      - § Obvious evidence of injury to the spine (cuts, punctures, bruises)
      - § Incontinence

Examination of the Spine

- Do not allow the patient to move.
- Examination
  - ☐ Roll patient onto his/her side
    - -Use 3-4 rescuers to keep the patient's spine immobilized
  - ☐ Palpate every vertebrae
  - ☐ Look for signs of a back injury

Clearing a C-Spine

- There are situations in the wilderness when determining if the cervical spine is free from injury is important.
- This might be seen when evacuation makes it essential.
- So when a significant mechanism of injury is present, a cervical spine is determined to be stable if:
  - ☐ There is no posterior midline cervical tenderness
  - ☐ There is no evidence of intoxication
  - ☐ The patient is alert and oriented to person, place, time, and event

☐ There is no focal neurological deficit

☐ There are no painful distracting injuries (e.g., long bone fracture)

A pneumonic for remember this is:

☐ C - Cervical midline tenderness

☐ S – Sensory motor deficit

☐ P – Pain or psychological distraction

☐ I – Intoxication

☐ N – Neurological deficit

☐ E – Events (MOI)

Treatment

Remember is it always better to over treat suspected spinal cord injuries ather than undertreat.

Start with manually stabilizing the head and cervical spine

☐ Keep the patient as still as possible

☐ Assure an airway (use jaw thrust if needed)

Check for circulation, sensation and motion in the extremities

Apply a cervical collar

Move patient to a backboard or rigid litter

EVACUATION GUIDELINES

Suspected skull fracture

Penetrating head wound

If a concussion is suspected then those displaying persistent vomiting, severe headache, amnesia of loss of consciousness

Anyone suspected of a vertebral body fracture

Anyone suspected of having a spinal cord injury

QUESTIONS

1. **Bleeding from head wounds should be treated with a bulky dressing because?**
   a) Bulky material is found more readily in the back country
   b) This type of dressing will absorb blood more readily
   c) It will help prevent bone fragments from pressing into the brain in the event that there is a skull fracture

2. **Regarding concussions:**
   a) All patients with suspected concussions should be evacuated
   b) It is defined as a physiologic injury to the brain
   c) Trauma to the skull is always seen.

3. **What is the Battle sign?**
   a) Swelling and black and blue around the eyes
   b) Redness and discoloration behind the ears

4. **Subdural hematomas:**
   a) Are usually from an artery and patients usually have symptoms quickly
   b) Are usually from a vein and patients usually have symptoms more slowly.

ANSWERS
1. c 2. b 3. b 4. b

CHAPTER 15

Heat-Induced Injuries

This chapter describes how to recognize and treat health conditions caused by a warm environment and how to help prevent these injuries.

Objectives:

- Be able to list factors that make someone susceptible to heat illness
- Be able to describe the etiology and management of victims with heat cramps and heat syncope
- Know the similarities and differences between heat exhaustion and heat stroke
- Discuss methods to help prevent heat-related illness
- Know methods of cooling, which method(s) is best in heat illness, and when to stop active cooling
- Be able to list evacuation guidelines for victims with heat illness

Case

During a long distance running event, three victims are brought to your first aid station:

Victim #1: A 27-year-old female "passed out" while standing at a hydration table, where she had stopped to drink some fluids. She wakes shortly after falling to the ground. She is alert and oriented to person, place, time, and event. She denies dizziness, nausea, or weakness and asks if she can continue running.

Victim #2: A 42-year-old male complains of severe spasms in his right calf muscle. He has been drinking large amounts of pure water throughout the day.

Victim #3: A 35-year-old is brought to the aid station by bystanders. They state that the victim was moving erratically and "just not acting right." The victim is obviously confused about the situation. He is covered with sweat and is agitated and warm to the touch.

1. What type of heat illness does each victim have?
2. How should each victim be managed?
3. Can any of these victims continue the race?
4. Who needs to be evacuated immediately?

DEHYDRATION

- Dehydration occurs when more water and fluids are exiting the body than are entering the body.
- 75% of the body is made up of water found inside cells, within blood vessels, and between cells.
- Survival in the wilderness requires a rather sophisticated water management system.
- Thirst indicates when a person needs to increase fluid intake.
- Although water is lost constantly throughout the day as we breathe, sweat, urinate, and defecate, we can replenish the water in our body by drinking fluids.
- The body can also shift water around to areas where it is more needed if dehydration begins to occur.
- The immediate causes of dehydration include not enough water, too much water loss, or some combination of the two.
- Sometimes it is not possible to consume enough while hiking or camping.
- Additional causes of dehydration include:
  - ☐ Diarrhea
  - ☐ Vomiting
  - ☐ Sweating
  - ☐ Diabetes
  - ☐ Frequent urination
  - ☐ Burns
  - ☐ Higher altitude

Symptoms of dehydration

The first symptoms of dehydration include headache, thirst, darker urine, and decreased urine production. Urine color is one of the best indicators of a person's hydration level - clear urine means you are well hydrated and darker urine means you are dehydrated.

As the condition progresses to moderate dehydration, symptoms include:

- ☐ Dry mouth
- ☐ Lethargy
- ☐ Muscle weakness
- ☐ Dizziness

Severe dehydration is characterized by extreme versions of symptoms mentioned above as well as:

- ☐ Lack of sweating
- ☐ Sunken eyes
- ☐ Shriveled and dry skin
- ☐ Low blood pressure
- ☐ Increased heart beat
- ☐ Fever
- ☐ Delirium
- ☐ Unconsciousness

Treatment of dehydration

Replenishing the fluid level in the body.

Consuming clear fluids such as water, clear broths, frozen water or sports drinks can do this.

People who are dehydrated should avoid drinks containing caffeine such as coffee, tea, and sodas

Prevention is really the most important treatment for dehydration.

Consuming plenty of fluids and foods that have high water content (such as fruits and vegetables) is essential to prevent dehydration.

HEAT AND THE BODY

The body produces heat in two ways the basic metabolic rate (BMR) and through exercise metabolism.

The body regulates temperature like a furnace. It is constantly producing heat and then dispersing it through various processes.

Heat can be lost through three processes called conduction, convection, radiation, and also evaporation (which uses all three.)

- ☐ Conduction is the process of losing heat through physical contact with another object or body. For example, if you were to sit on a metal chair, the heat from your body would transfer to the cold metal chair.
- ☐ Convection is the process of losing heat through the movement of air or water molecules across the skin. The use of a fan to cool off the body is one example of convection. The amount of heat loss from convection is dependent upon the airflow or in aquatic exercise, the water flow over the skin. This is where the wind-chill factor takes place.

- ☐ Radiation is a form of heat loss through infrared rays. This involves the transfer of heat from one object to another, with no physical contact involved. For example, the sun transfers heat to the earth through radiation.
- ☐ The last process of heat loss is evaporation. Evaporation is the process of losing heat through the conversion of water to gas (evaporation of sweat). It utilizes convection, conduction and radiation. In order for evaporation to work, sweat on the skin must evaporate and just drip off onto the floor.
- There is no such thing as 'cold.' We commonly refer to something being cold, but really what we mean is that this object just has less heat.
- Heat is transferred from one object to another, not cold. And crazy as it seems, if you hold ice up to your skin, you are not transferring cold into the body, you are transferring heat out of the body.
- If the ability to remove heat from the body is lost, then the body temperature will rise and heat illnesses will occur.

RISK FACTORS FOR HEAT ILLNESS

Medical Conditions

- Heart disease
- Dehydration
- Vomiting
- Diarrhea
- Fever
- Previous heat exhaustion or heat stroke

Environmental Conditions

- Exercise in a hot environment, particularly if there is high humidity
- Lack of air conditioning or proper ventilation
- Inappropriate clothing (occlusive, heavy, or vapor-impermeable)
- Lack of acclimatization
- Decreased fluid intake
- Hot environments (inside of tents or autos in the sun, hot tubs, saunas)

Drugs & Toxins

- Alcohol
- Antihistamines (including Benadryl)
- Certain motion sickness medications, such as meclizine and Dramamine
- Cocaine, amphetamines, and other stimulant drugs

Other Risk Factors

- Salt and/or water depletion
- Obesity

TYPES OF HEAT ILLNESS

Heat Cramps

Heat cramps occur when significant salt and water losses are replaced with solutions not containing sufficient salt (sodium chloride or NaCl). Inadequate salt repletion can eventually lead to involuntary contraction of skeletal muscles. Signs of heat cramps include the following:

- Brief, intermittent, involuntary contractions of skeletal muscles
- Cramps that most commonly involve the calves, but may occur in any muscle
- Cramps that usually only occur in a single muscle or muscle group and are quite painful
- The victim with heat cramps will classically give a history of the following:
  - ☐ Prolonged activity in a hot environment
  - ☐ Attempted hydration, typically with a non-electrolyte containing solution, such as plain water
  - ☐ Poor salt/electrolyte intake

Treatment

- Mild cases
  - ☐ Oral salt replacement.
  - ☐ This can be easily made with ¼ to ½ teaspoon of table salt added to a quart of water.
- Severe cases
  - ☐ If not responding to the above treatment, the individual may require intravenous fluids and should be evacuated.

Heat Syncope

Syncope is the medical term for "passing out," usually a brief loss of consciousness. Heat syncope typically occurs when a dehydrated individual stands in a hot environment for an extended period. With standing, blood pools in the legs, decreasing the amount of blood that returns to the heart. This, in combination with dehydration and dilated blood vessels from the hot environment, can decrease blood flow to the brain and cause the individual to faint. Prior to actually losing consciousness, the victim may have the following signs and symptoms:

- Lightheadedness
- Vertigo / dizziness
- Dimming or graying of vision
- Restlessness
- Nausea
- Yawning

These symptoms and the actual loss of consciousness usually resolve once the victim is horizontal, as this facilitates redistribution of blood from the legs back to the brain.

Treatment

- The loss of consciousness should be brief, on the order of several seconds up to two minutes.
- Treatment to improve blood flow to the brain should be instituted.
  - ☐ Lay the victim flat on their back (supine).
  - ☐ Elevate the feet to improve venous return back to the heart.
  - ☐ Loosen tight or constrictive clothing.
  - ☐ Remove from direct sunlight.
  - ☐ Move to a cool area if possible.
  - ☐ Have the victim drink fluids once consciousness is regained.
- ■ Assess the victim for other injuries that may have resulted from the fall

Heat Exhaustion

Heat exhaustion is a form of heat illness that results from a significant heat stress. Heat exhaustion is part of a continuum of heat illnesses that progress to heat stroke.

Symptoms

- Weakness
- Lightheadedness
- Fatigue
- Nausea with or without vomiting
- Headache
- Thirst
- Rapid heartbeat and breathing
- Profuse sweating

Treatment

- Cease all physical activity.
- Replace fluids and electrolytes liberally. With heat exhaustion, oral hydration as discussed below is appropriate.
- Remove the victim from direct sunlight into a cool, shaded area.
- Loosen restrictive clothing.
- If the victim is hyperthermic (> 38 degrees C or 100.4 degrees F), take active cooling measures. In the wilderness, there are limited resources to actively cool a victim.
- The best way to cool a hyperthermic victim is through **evaporative cooling**.
  - ☐ Remove most of the victim's clothing and make them "sopping wet" with tepid (room temperature) water. While it may seem paradoxical to cool a hyperthermic victim with warm water, the warm temperature of the water helps to prevent shivering and keeps the skin blood vessels dilated, which allows for heat exchange. Cold water might lead to shivering and constriction of the blood vessels in the skin. However, if only cold water is available, use it.

☐ Fan the victim with anything that will increase air movement across the skin. This air flow will result in evaporation of water from the skin, which cools the victim.

☐ Shivering will increase core body temperature and should be avoided.

Oral hydration should adhere to the following guidelines:

☐ Cool/cold water or sports drink

☐ Beverage should not exceed 6% carbohydrate content. Increased carbohydrate content inhibits fluid absorption. You can dilute most sports drinks with water to achieve a better concentration.

☐ A general rule is that every pound lost to sweat should be replenished with 500 mL or two cups of fluid.

☐ The treatment goal for mild heat exhaustion should be 1 to 2 liters of oral fluids over two to four hours.

Heat Stroke

Heat stroke is a true medical emergency that is classically defined by the following:

☐ Severe hyperthermia (core temperature > 40°C or 104°F)

☐ Central nervous system (CNS) disturbances such as alteration in the level of consciousness, confusion, or seizures

☐ Lack of active sweating

However, experience has shown that waiting for the appearance of these three symptoms is too strict and may delay critical treatment.

Any person who has any of the following symptoms in a hot environment should be treated as having heat stroke:

☐ Unsteady gait (often one of the first manifestations of heat stroke)

☐ Irritability

☐ Confusion

☐ Combativeness

☐ Bizarre behavior

☐ Seizures

☐ Hallucinations

☐ Coma (very late finding)

■ Diminished or lack of sweating is classically associated with heat stroke; however, it is typically a late finding and cannot be relied upon to make an accurate diagnosis. Typically, heat stroke victims will be covered in sweat until very late stages of the illness.

The key to treatment and prevention of heat stroke is in the understanding that heat exhaustion and heat stroke are not separate entities, but are a continuum of the same illness. The onset of any alteration in mental status should alert the wilderness medicine provider that a victim is suffering from significant heat illness.

Treatment

The primary goal of treatment for heat stroke is to facilitate rapid cooling, which can be accomplished by evaporative cooling as discussed previously.

Additionally, one may place ice packs or cold compresses in areas where large blood vessels are superficial, such as the neck, axilla, groin, and scalp.

Most persons will not have a rectal thermometer to measure temperature. However, it may be used when one is available:

☐ The goal of treatment is to drop the temperature to below 40°C (104° F) as rapidly as possible.

☐ Active cooling efforts should be discontinued around 39°C (102.2°F) to avoid overshoot to a condition of hypothermia, which can occur with very successful cooling efforts.

PREVENTION

Hydration

Drink at least four to eight ounces of water or sports drink every 15-20 minutes during mild to moderate physical activity, depending on the ambient environmental temperature and humidity.

Hydrate with a goal of clear urine instead of a fixed amount of intake.

Consume salt-containing foods or add salt to water if exposed to heat for time periods greater than two to three hours, especially if using only water for hydration.

To make a salt solution, add one-fourth to one-half teaspoon of table salt to a liter of fluid. Flavored drinks that are cold are more palatable.

Most commercially available sports drinks should be diluted with an equal amount of water for ideal electrolyte concentration.

Heat Dissipation

Wear loose-fitting clothing that will allow for air circulation and increased evaporation.

Avoid direct sunlight when possible and wear light-colored clothing.

Douse with cool fluids or cool misting spray frequently.

Heat Acclimatization

Heat acclimatization decreases the incidence of heat injuries and improves performance in hot environments. The general guidelines for acclimatization include the following:

Adults should gradually increase the time and intensity of activity in a hot environment over 7 to 10 days.

Children and elderly people require 10 to 14 days to maximize acclimatization.

Those who are from temperate or cold climates and will be traveling into a hot environment can acclimatize by going into a sauna or steam room for increasing amounts of time each day, beginning 7 to 10 days before making the trip.

De-acclimatization usually occurs within one to two weeks of being removed from the hot environment. In such a situation, acclimatization must be repeated if necessary.

EVACUATION GUIDELINES

A victim who suffers a fainting episode thought to be heat-related should only have brief loss of consciousness and recover quickly. Any victim who endures a prolonged loss of consciousness, persistent pre-syncope signs and symptoms upon awakening, more than one episode of passing out, or signs of heat stroke should be evacuated.

A victim with severe heat cramps that do not respond to oral salt solutions, or a victim who suffers diffuse and multiple cramps should also be considered for evacuation, depending on the situation.

Heat exhaustion victims *may not* need to be evacuated:

☐ As long as the victim can adequately be protected from the environment.

- ☐ In mild cases, close observation in the field for development of heat stroke, as well as cessation of activities for 24-48 hours, is recommended.
- ☐ If the victim develops behavioral changes, records a temperature above 39°C (102.2°F), or has a fainting episode while under observation, he should be considered a potential heat stroke victim and be evacuated immediately.
- Heat stroke is a serious medical emergency, so any victim with signs or symptoms of heat stroke should be evacuated as soon as possible.

QUESTIONS

1. **All of the following increase the risk of heat illness except:**
   a) Heart disease
   b) History of heat injury
   c) Diarrhea
   d) Alcohol
   e) All of the above increase the risk of heat injury

2. **Heat cramps are most likely to occur in which victim?**
   a) A runner on a hot day drinking water alternated with a sports drink
   b) A runner on a hot day not rehydrating with anything
   c) A runner on a hot day drinking 20 oz of water per hour for several hours
   d) A runner on a hot day drinking 20 oz of water per hour for two hours

3. **Which one of the following is the most important difference between heat stroke and heat exhaustion?**
   a) Core body temperature
   b) The presence or absence of sweating
   c) The presence of vomiting
   d) Altered mental status

4. **Which one of the following is the most effective way to cool a victim under most conditions?**
   a) Cold water immersion
   b) Cold water evaporative cooling
   c) Ice packs to the axilla/groin
   d) Tepid water evaporative cooling

5. **Acclimatization to a hot environment should take how long for the average adult?**
   a) 1-3 days
   b) 4-6 days
   c) 7-10 days
   d) 11-14 days

ANSWERS
1. e   2. c   3. d   4. d   5. c

CHAPTER 16

Hypothermia and Cold Injuries

This chapter discusses cold-induced injuries and illnesses.

Objectives:

- Understand the mechanisms by which the body loses and gains heat
- Recognize and diagnose hypothermia, frostbite, and other cold-related injuries
- Understand the principles of backcountry treatment of cold injuries
- Learn about prevention of these conditions when exposed to cold weather

Case

While on a cold weather backpacking trip, you come upon a solo hiker who became lost and now has been outside much longer than expected. He is shivering uncontrollably and appears to be confused.

1. What are the ways that heat is lost from the body?
2. Should he be evacuated?
3. What is the severity of his hypothermia?
4. How should you treat him?

HYPOTHERMIA

Mild hypothermia

- Defined as a core body temperature ranging from 32 to 35°C (90.0 to 95°F)
- Signs of mild hypothermia include the following:
  - ☐ Pale and cold skin secondary to blood vessel constriction
  - ☐ Uncontrollable shivering as the body attempts to produce heat
  - ☐ Varying degrees of confusion, unsteady gait, and disorientation
  - ☐ Frequent urination
  - ☐ Elevated pulse and breathing rate

Moderate hypothermia

- Defined as a core temperature ranging from 28 to 32°C (82.0 to 90.0°F)
- Signs of moderate hypothermia include the following:
  - ☐ Decreased rates of blood pressure, pulse, and breathing
  - ☐ Severe confusion as well as dilated pupils and muscle rigidity
- Unless rewarming is possible, the patient will eventually cool to ambient temperature and die.

Severe hypothermia

- Defined as a core temperature below 28°C (82.0°F)
- Signs of severe hypothermia include the following:
  - ☐ Deep coma with dilated pupils and muscular rigidity
  - ☐ Pulse may be as low as 10-20 beats per minute and may be difficult to feel.
  - ☐ People in severe hypothermia often appear to be dead.

Treatment

- The most important consideration in treating hypothermia is removing the patient from the situation that caused them to become hypothermic.
- If a patient cannot be evacuated, attempts should be made to get him or her to a shelter that is out of cold, wet, and windy conditions that may precipitate further heat loss.
- Wet clothes should be removed, and patients should be wrapped in dry blankets if possible.
- Anything that can be done to help rewarm the patient will be helpful, such as sitting them by a fire or giving them warm liquids. It is important however to avoid beverages such as alcohol or heavily caffeinated drinks, which may worsen hypothermia.
- In a rescue situation, it is important to remember the premise that "no one is dead until they are warm and dead." People suffering from severe hypothermia may be severely comatose, though alive, and will recover with proper medical care.

The following are specific recommendations for treatment of the different levels of hypothermia in the field. However, keep in mind that field treatment of hypothermia is notoriously difficult, and arrangements should begin for evacuation as soon as it is determined that the patient cannot actively rewarm himself or herself:

Mild hypothermia

Remove the patient from the elements and move into shelter to avoid further heat loss.

Undress the individual completely, then dress them in dry clothes and wrap them in blankets taking special care to cover the head and neck to avoid heat loss.

Warmed, sweetened beverages may be helpful.

Limited exercise may generate some heat (this is not advised in moderate and severe hypothermia).

Moderate hypothermia (in addition to the treatments mentioned above)

Apply mild heat to the head, neck, chest, armpits and groin of the patient using hot water bottles, wrapped commercial heating pads, or warm moist towels.

If conditions prohibit the use of a fire to warm fluids, chemical heaters such as those found in military "meals ready to eat" can be used for this purpose.

Severe hypothermia

It is important to consider that patients suffering from this condition may exhibit altered mental status if they are still conscious. Therefore, it is vital to ignore pleas of "Leave me alone, I'm okay" because these individuals are in serious trouble.

If evacuation is not possible, place the patient in a pre-warmed sleeping bag with one to two people. Skin-to-skin contact is very important to promote transfer of warmth to the patient through conduction. It is particularly useful to initiate skin-to-skin contact in regions of the body with large surface area and where major blood vessels are more superficial, such as the chest and neck areas.

Inhalation of warm, humidified air into the lungs can aid in rewarming key areas of the body such as the head, neck, and thorax.

Care must be taken in handling patients suffering from this condition as extremely cold core temperatures can cause irritability of the heart muscle. Even a small bump can cause the heart to fibrillate and stop beating effectively.

Above all else, it is crucial to closely monitor individuals suffering from this condition. Remember that severe hypothermia may mimic other medical conditions and may mimic death as well.

Prevention

The single most important aspect in hypothermia prevention is adequate preparation.
- ☐ Maintain awareness of weather conditions.
- ☐ Bring the proper gear.
- ☐ Design a contingency plan in case the worst should occur.
- ☐ Remember also that the weather does not need to be sub-zero in order for hypothermia to set in.

Should the unexpected occur and you are faced with this situation, the following is a list of things that can be done to help prevent hypothermia:

- ☐ Find or create a shelter.

- ☐ Cover exposed areas of the body.
- ☐ Wear several loosely fitting layers of clothing.
- ☐ Conserve, share, and create warmth.
- ☐ Share body heat.
- ☐ Increase heat production through voluntary muscle movement.
- ☐ Consume warm beverages and food.
- ☐ Build a fire.
- ☐ Monitor for signs and symptoms of hypothermia.

FROSTBITE

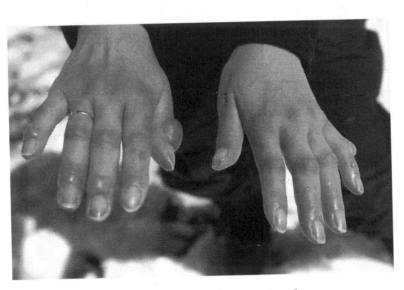

Figure 16.1 Frostbitten Hands

Frostbite is the freezing of skin that may involve deeper tissues.

Frostbite is divided into degrees first through fourth and superficial through deep in a manner similar to burns.

First- and second-degree frostbite are considered to be superficial and typically heal well with minor long-term consequences, while third-degree and fourth-degree frostbite are deeper and associated with very significant permanent damage and tissue loss.

The following is a description of the different degrees of frostbite:

First Degree (Superficial)

This involves the superficial layers of skin.

The skin appears pale and white while frozen and is numb to the touch.

With rewarming, there will be pain and redness of the involved area.

After rewarming, the area will be swollen and continue to be red for a period of hours.

Second Degree (Superficial)

This involves deeper layers of the skin.

The skin appears pale and white while frozen and is numb to the touch.

- With rewarming, there will be pain and redness of the involved area.
- After rewarming, the area will be swollen and continue to be red for a period of hours.
- In addition to the redness, the skin will develop blisters over the area of involvement. These blisters will be filled with a clear fluid.

Third Degree (Deep)

- This involves complete freezing of the skin and tissue layers under the skin.
- The skin appears pale and white while frozen and is numb to the touch.
- With rewarming, there will be pain, redness and swelling of the involved area.
- After rewarming, the area will be swollen and continue to be red for a period of hours to days.
- In addition to the redness, the skin will develop blisters over the area of involvement. These blisters will be filled with a bloody fluid.

Fourth Degree (Deep)

- This involves the skin and much deeper tissues including muscle, tendon, and bone.
- The area of involvement appears pale and white while frozen.
- Numb to the touch, the skin has a "chunk of wood" type of consistency.
- With rewarming, there will be significant pain, redness and swelling of the involved area.
- After rewarming, the area will be swollen and continue to be red for a period of hours to days.
- In addition to the redness, the skin will develop blisters over the area of involvement. These blisters will be filled with a bloody fluid.
- Mottled skin with bluish discoloration forms a deep, dry, black crusted lesion.

Treatment

- In general, all frostbite should be treated in a medical facility by health care providers.
  - ☐ Thawing of a frozen body part is a very painful process that usually requires narcotic pain medications and other medications such as antibiotics and anti-inflammatory agents.
  - ☐ An inappropriate or poorly done thawing process will cause the patient more harm.
- Prior to rewarming, treat the patient with ibuprofen 400 mg if they have no allergy to it.
- The primary treatment is rapid rewarming in a controlled manner.
  - ☐ This should only occur when there is no chance of the person refreezing the area of involvement.
    - Refreezing of a previously thawed frostbitten body part will result in a significant increase in the amount of damage that occurs.
    - A failure to rewarm in a rapid manner will increase tissue damage.
- The optimal method of rewarming is to place the affected body part into gently circulated water that has been warmed to 40-42°C (104-108°F).
  - ☐ This should be done for at least 15-30 minutes or until skin regains pliability and returns to its normal color.
  - ☐ A good rule of thumb is to heat the water until it approximates the temperature of a hot tub.
  - ☐ The temperature must be closely monitored with a thermometer. If it is too hot, it will burn the skin, which will worsen the injury. If it is too cool, it will delay thawing, which will worsen the injury.
- Additional measures that may be taken in the wilderness setting include the following:
  - ☐ Remove all wet clothing and replace it with dry clothes.
  - ☐ Remove any tight or constrictive clothing.

- ☐ If possible, wrap the involved area with clean gauze. If the frostbite involves the hands or feet, separate the fingers toes with dry gauze in addition to wrapping the hand/foot.
- ☐ Elevate the extremity to reduce swelling.
- ☐ Pad the skin with cotton or gauze.
- ☐ Treat pain with medicines such as acetaminophen and ibuprofen.

DO NOTS OF FROSTBITE TREATMENT

- ☐ Do not attempt thawing by heating with dry heat such as a fire. The fact that the temperature is not controlled may lead to delay in thawing but may also burn the area as the area is numb.
- ☐ Do not thaw the area if there is any chance that the area will refreeze. If a body part undergoes freezing again soon after being rewarmed the extent of the injury is much worse than if there was just a delay in the thawing. An example is the person with the frostbitten foot in the wilderness. It is better to have that person walk out on the frozen foot than to risk a refreezing injury, if it is possible.
- ☐ Do not rub the area when it is frozen or thawing as that will worsen the injury.
- ☐ Do not rub the area with snow. This is an old recommendation that was proven to be harmful in the 1950s.

Prevention

- Covering susceptible areas of skin with properly fitting dry clothing and footgear is essential during prolonged exposure to cold weather. To this end, a waterproof bag containing an extra pair of socks and undergarments may come in handy.
- Maintain a good diet and stay well hydrated.
- Consumption of alcohol and smoking cigarettes may also contribute to frostbite and should therefore be avoided.
- In extreme situations, putting one's hand or feet in his or her partner's armpits may provide some added warmth.
- Continuous movement, including frequent contraction and relaxation of extremities, may also be helpful.

FROSTNIP

- Frostnip is a cold injury to the skin, but there is not the actual tissue freezing that occurs in frostbite.
- It is the result of prolonged skin exposure to cold temperatures.
- Frostnip can be a **precursor to frostbite** and should therefore be taken seriously.
- Signs of frostnip include the following:
  - ☐ The affected area will be red and swollen, but the skin will stay soft and pliable.
  - ☐ Numbness and tingling are possible but should resolve after rewarming.
  - ☐ Frostnip only has mild pain when rewarming.
  - ☐ Pain and skin cracking are possible in areas that are repeatedly frostnipped, potentially leading to infection.
  - ☐ Areas that are most commonly affected include fingers, toes, ears, and cheeks.

Treatment

- Rewarm the injured area using water, fire, or another heat source.
- Take care not to rub frostnipped areas as this may promote tissue damage.

■ Unlike frostbite, these injuries should always be rewarmed even if still exposed to a cold environment since the tissue has not yet been damaged and will only become damaged if the process is allowed to continue.

CHILBLAINS

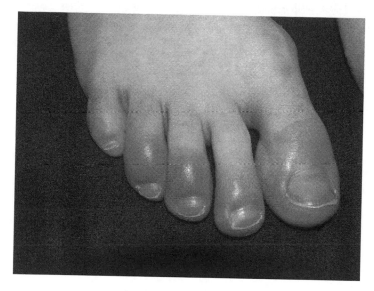

Figure 16.2 Chilblains

■ Chilblains occur at temperatures from 0-15°C (0-59°F) and result from an abnormal reaction of the body to the cold.
■ Several different conditions have been linked to the formation of chilblains including the following:
  ☐ Poor circulation
  ☐ Rapid rewarming
  ☐ Damp living conditions
  ☐ Sudden exposure to cold water
■ Signs of chilblains include the following:
  ☐ Itchy, red or purple bumps on the skin that emerge over the course of several hours and can become very painful.
  ☐ Common places where chilblains occur include the backs and sides of fingers and toes, lower extremities, heels, nose, and ears.
  ☐ Blistering, ulceration, and infection are possible, but they generally resolve spontaneously over the course of one to two weeks.

Treatment

■ Treatment generally consists of elevation, gentle rewarming, and covering the area with a dry bandage.
■ Diphenhydramine (Benadryl) may be helpful to relieve the itching.

Prevention

- Certain groups of people predisposed to chilblains include children, the elderly, and people with poor blood flow to the arms, hands, legs and feet.
- Keep legs and feet warm with leg warmers or wool socks.
- Avoid smoking, as this causes constriction of the blood vessels.
- Wear warm, waterproof gloves if working in wet environments.
- Exercise and acclimatize before prolonged exposure to a cold environment.
- Soak hands in warm water and then dry to promote dilation of blood vessels.

IMMERSION FOOT

- Immersion foot, also known as trench foot, occurs as the result of several days of exposure to water at non-freezing temperatures. Ambient temperatures generally consistent with immersion foot range from 0-10°C (32-50°F).
- Signs and symptoms of immersion foot include the following:
  - [ ] Redness followed by bluish discoloration and mottling
  - [ ] Swelling
  - [ ] Numbness, tingling, and pain
  - [ ] The patient's foot may appear to be shiny, and the patient may describe the foot as feeling "wooden" in severe cases.
  - [ ] Although uncommon, the development of blisters, ulcers, and even gangrene are possible.

Treatment

- Most cases of immersion foot resolve spontaneously over the course of several weeks provided they are removed from the offending conditions.
- Acutely, the affected area should be kept warm and dry.

Prevention

- Keep feet warm and dry by changing wet socks and boot / shoes as often as possible.
- Allow feet to air dry whenever possible.
- Frequently inspect feet for signs and symptoms of this condition.

EVACUATION GUIDELINES

Hypothermia

- Mild – Evacuation is a judgment call. If the patient can be removed from the elements, can be dressed in dry clothing, and can adequately rewarm himself or herself, evacuation is not absolutely necessary.
- Moderate and severe require evacuation.

Frostbite

- Everything except first-degree frostbite should be evacuated from the field.

Frostnip, chilblains, and immersion foot

- These do not generally require evacutation

QUESTIONS

1. **In which degree of hypothermia is uncontrollable shivering a feature?**
   a) Mild hypothermia
   b) Moderate hypothermia
   c) Severe hypothermia

2. **Which one of the following is not a step that should be taken to prevent further hypothermia in the victim who is cold?**
   a) Getting the patient to shelter
   b) Using body heat
   c) Drinking warm beverages
   d) Smoking cigarettes
   e) Removing wet clothing

3. **Which one of the following is an important medication that you must administer to the patient who has frostbite before they undergo rapid rewarming of the frostbitten body part?**
   a) Acetaminophen (Tylenol)
   b) Epinephrine (EpiPen)
   c) Heparin
   d) Ibuprofen
   e) Nitroglycerin

4. **Which degree of frostbite is associated with full-thickness skin involvement in addition to muscle and tendon involvement with hemorrhagic bullae?**
   a) First degree
   b) Second degree
   c) Third degree
   d) Fourth degree

5. **When should frostbite not be treated in the field with rewarming?**
   a) If the patient will be promptly evacuated
   b) If the patient is diabetic
   c) If there is a possibility of refreezing

6. How does frostnip differ from frostbite?
   a) There is no ice crystal formation in frostnip
   b) Permanent damage occurs, but it is very minor with frostnip but not first-degree frostbite
   c) Frostnip only involves the surface of the skin and frostbite goes down to the muscle
   d) Frostbite has hemorrhagic bullae, whereas frostnip has white to clear bullae

ANSWERS

1. a   2. d   3. d   4. d   5. c   6. a

CHAPTER 17

Infectious Disease

This chapter will train you on infectious diseases that may occur in the wilderness setting.

Objectives:

- Understand the incidence and epidemiology of infectious diseases as they pertain to wilderness travel.
- Describe the most common gastrointestinal infections that may occur in the wilderness and be able to describe their clinical presentation, treatment, and prevention.
- Describe the clinical presentation, treatment, and prevention of malaria.
- Describe two ways to ascertain the risk of malaria on a proposed trip and the best way to find the correct preventive medication.
- Explain the appropriate treatment and management of a person who sustains a bite from an animal that is worrisome for rabies.
- Describe various tick-borne diseases in terms of their clinical presentation and treatment.

DISESASES AFFECTING THE GASTROINTESTINAL SYSTEM

- Gastrointestinal (stomach – intestinal) illnesses are the most commonly encountered infectious diseases in the wilderness.
- Up to 50% of wilderness travelers are affected by gastrointestinal diseases, mainly diarrhea.
- The vast majority of these diseases are passed by fecal-oral (stool to mouth) transmission through contaminated food or water.
- Among the most common organisms causing symptomatic disease are *Staphylococcus aureus*, *Salmonella* species, enterotoxigenic *E. coli*, *Campylobacter jejuni*, *Giardia lamblia*, and viruses.
- Most diarrheal illnesses are categorized as either dysenteric or non-dysenteric. Organisms causing non-dysenteric gastroenteritis usually colonize the inner lining of the small bowel. This results in a non-bloody, high volume, watery diarrhea. Organisms causing dysentery usually invade the ileum and colon causing a lower volume, bloody, and leukocyte-containing diarrhea.

Staphylococcal Enteritis

Pathophysiology

- Acute gastroenteritis may result from eating food contaminated by a toxin produced by *Staphylococcus aureus*.
- *Staphylococcus* colonizes human skin; food may easily become contaminated during its preparation.
- While the bacteria can grow in any food, those that are high in protein, such as mayonnaise, milk, cream, custard, and meat products, are most conducive to overgrowth of *Staphylococcus*.
- If contaminated food is left unrefrigerated for several hours, as is commonly encountered in the wilderness, the bacteria are allowed to multiply and the enterotoxin is produced.
  - ☐ The toxin is heat resistant and cannot be eliminated by reheating or boiling contaminated food.
  - ☐ Upon ingestion, the toxin acts on the gastrointestinal tract to cause the acute gastroenteritis characteristic of the disease.

Clinical presentation

- Staphylococcal gastroenteritis (the medical name given to describe the stomach flu) is characterized by acute onset of nausea, severe vomiting, mild diarrhea, and abdominal cramps.
- Symptoms may occur within one to six hours after ingestion of contaminated food, with an average time of onset of three hours.
- The etiology of food poisoning may be seen when multiple victims have vomiting and diarrhea after consuming the same food.
- Staphylococcal food poisoning is self limited, and symptoms typically resolve within twenty-four hours.

Treatment

- Treatment is supportive and based upon symptoms, with fluid and electrolyte replacement as the primary goal.
- Anti-nausea medications may be used.

Antibiotic therapy is ineffective and unnecessary because the toxin is pre-formed and cannot be neutralized.

Prevention

Staphylococcal enteritis may be avoided by using proper hygiene and sanitation with food preparation.
Hand sanitation with alcohol gels or hand washing with soap and water is essential.
Food prepared in the wilderness must be consumed immediately after preparation, and leftovers should be disposed of properly.

Non-dysenteric gastroenteritis

Pathophysiology

Acute, watery diarrhea associated with wilderness travel domestically or internationally may be caused by a variety of organisms.
Enterotoxigenic *E. coli* is by far the most common cause in developing areas and accounts for 30% – 70% of "traveler's diarrhea."
Viral gastroenteritis is the most common cause in the developing world, with Norwalk and rotaviruses being the most common agents.
Worldwide, *Vibrio cholera* accounts for a significant number of deaths even though it is rare in travelers due to large inoculum required for infection. This is due to its characteristic explosive "rice water stools" that can be produced at a rate of up to one liter per hour leading to massive fluid loss and severe dehydration.
In general, these agents produce a toxin, which causes water to get into the intestines which causes diarrhea resulting in the secretion of water and electrolytes into the intestinal lumen.
These enteric pathogens are typically spread by fecal-oral contamination, with contaminated food and water as the most common vehicles for transmission.

Clinical Presentation

Symptoms include profuse watery diarrhea, abdominal cramping, nausea and vomiting, and malaise.
Adults are usually afebrile, but low-grade fever may be present.
Incubation times from ingestion to clinical presentation usually range from 12 to 72 hours.

Treatment

Non-dysenteric diarrhea typically runs a self-limited course with symptoms resolving within one week.
The mainstay of treatment is replacement of fluid and electrolyte losses.
Oral intake should at least approximate fluid losses in stool.
A variety of oral rehydration solutions may be used:
□ U.S. Public Heath Service Formula:
   – Glass One
      ▪ 8 oz fruit juice
      ▪ ½ teaspoon baking soda
      ▪ ½ teaspoon honey or corn syrup
   – Glass Two
      ▪ 8 oz water
      ▪ 1 pinch table salt

- □ Drink equal amounts from each glass alternating between the two.
- WHO (World Health Organization) Oral Rehydration Solution may be purchased as small packets in most developing countries.
  - □ Add one packet to a liter of disinfected water.
  - □ For a WHO ORS equivalent, add the following ingredients to one liter of clean water:
    - – 3/4 teaspoon of salt (two finger pinch)
    - – ½ teaspoon baking soda (one finger pinch)
    - – 2-3 tablespoons of sugar (three finger scoop)
    - – ¼ teaspoon potassium chloride salt substitute (small pinch)--if available
- Sports drinks such as Gatorade or Power Ade may be used if diluted to half strength with clean water.
  - □ Only disinfected or bottled water and juices should be used.
  - □ Urine volume and color should be monitored as an indicator of hydration status. As a general rule, the clearer the urine the better hydrated the individual is.
- Antidiarrheal medications
  - □ Loperamide (Imodium) may be used with noninvasive gastroenteritis to reduce cramping and fluid losses.
  - □ Bismuth subsalicylate (Pepto-Bismol) is an effective treatment for travel-related diarrhea and has comparable treatment results to antibiotic therapy in mild to moderate cases. An appropriate adult dose of bismuth subsalicylate is 2 tablespoons or 2 tablets PO every hour up to eight doses in 24 hours.
- More severe cases of travel-related gastroenteritis may warrant empiric antibiotic therapy prescribed by a physician. The CDC recommends antibiotics if patients experience three or more episodes of diarrhea in an eight-hour period.

Bacterial Dysentery

Pathophysiology

- Invasive bacterial infections of the intestines produce more severe symptoms, including bloody diarrhea and fever.
- Up to 15% of travel related diarrhea is due to dysentery.
- Causative organisms include *Salmonella, Shigella, Campylobacter*, enterohemorrhagic *E. coli, Yersinia enterocolitica*, and *Aeromonas hydrophilia*.
- Most organisms causing dysentery are spread by a fecal-oral (stools) route mainly through contaminated food and water.
  - □ *Salmonella* species are widespread and are commonly found in raw eggs, poultry and meat.
  - □ Domestic animals and pets such as dogs, cats, birds, turtles and lizards are also common carriers of *Salmonella*.
  - □ *Shigella* is highly contagious and is usually transmitted from the hands of the last person to handle food and water contaminated with fecal matter. It is easily spread from person to person as ingestion of only a few organisms can cause infection.
  - □ *Campylobacter* is a very common contaminant of natural water supplies and is also common in unprocessed milk and uncooked meat, such as raw poultry products.
  - □ Enterohemorrhagic *E. coli* is also transmitted in contaminated food and water, particularly undercooked meats such as hamburger.
  - □ *Aeromonas hydrophilia* is spread through contaminated water and is more common in children.
  - □ Patients with a history of prior antibiotic use may develop overgrowth of *Clostridium difficile* resulting in pseudomembranous enterocolitis.

Clinical Presentation

- Acute onset of severe, intermittent abdominal cramps followed by diarrhea that may be copious, watery, and foul smelling.
- Blood and pus may be present in stools.
- Fever, often as high as 104° F (40° C), is a distinguishing feature as compared to noninvasive diarrhea.
- Headache and muscle aches are often present and vomiting may be minimal.
- The patient may experience severe abdominal pain and tenderness, especially in the lower abdomen.
- Rebound tenderness and guarding may be present on physical exam.
- Symptoms of bacteremia and sepsis may develop, especially in association with *Salmonella* and *Shigella* infections. These microbes are motile, increasing their chance of reaching an individual's bloodstream.
- Incubation periods vary from 8 hours to 8 days (longer in *C. difficile* colitis) and symptoms may persist from 1-10 days.

Treatment

- Fluid replacement with oral rehydration is again the most important aspect of treatment.
- Antibacterial medications as prescribed by a physician can be used in serious cases.
- Antidiarrheal medications such as loperamide (Imodium) or Lomotil are usually not used in the treatment of dysentery.
  - *The traditional teaching is that these medications should generally be avoided as they may allow for retention of the toxic bacteria.*
  - *However, voluminous or frequent diarrhea is generally terrible with most wilderness activities, so these medicines are more commonly used in this setting.*
- Bismuth subsalicylate (Pepto-Bismol) may be used safely in cases of dysentery, but it slows absorption of oral antibiotic medications.

Protozoal Causes of Diarrhea

- Common protozoal causes of gastroenteritis include *Giardia lamblia*, *Entamoeba histolytica*, *Cryptosporidium*, and *Cyclospora*.
- All are transmitted via the fecal-oral route, mainly in contaminated water and food.
- Protozoal infections can result in chronic diarrhea, but symptoms vary widely from asymptomatic disease to acute dysentery.

Giardiasis

Pathophysiology

- *Giardia lamblia* is a single-celled parasite that exists in a cyst form and a trophozoite form.
- Symptomatic disease is caused by the trophozoite.
- Infected individuals and animals pass the cyst form in stools. These cysts can survive in the environment for three months or longer.
- Beaver, deer, dogs, cattle, sheep, and rodents are common carriers of *Giardia*, and many natural water sources may have *Giardia* cysts present despite being in remote or "pristine" locations.

Drinking contaminated water is the primary source of infection with an infectious dose being as low as 10-25 cysts.

However, many individuals remain completely asymptomatic after exposure to *Giardia*, even in high concentrations.

The disease may also be transmitted in a direct person-to-person manner if proper hygiene is not observed.

Clinical Presentation

Incubation time is one to three weeks after ingestion, so many travelers may develop symptoms well after returning home.

Diarrhea is the most common feature of giardiasis and is present in up to 90% of symptomatic cases.

The severity of diarrhea varies and may result in mild to moderate amounts of foul smelling soft stool, but it can be copious and explosive.

A characteristic "rotten egg" odor is associated with the intestinal gas and feces.

Other symptoms include malaise, bloating, abdominal cramping, nausea, and occasionally vomiting and low-grade fever.

Untreated, symptoms typically last 7-10 days, but chronic diarrhea (> 2 weeks) may develop and can have a cyclical pattern of worsening symptoms every few weeks.

Treatment

A treatment regimen of antiparasitic drugs is used to properly treat *Giardia*. Some cases of giardiasis may be resistant and require multi-drug therapy. No single medication is effective in all cases.

Amebiasis

Pathophysiology

Amebiasis is caused by *Entamoeba histolytica,* a very common parasite found in water supplies around the world.

It is particularly prevalent in tropical countries.

The organism exists in two forms: a cyst and a trophozoite form with the cyst form being excreted in stool.

☐ The cysts are transmitted through fecal-oral contamination of food and water, or through direct contact with an infected person.

☐ Ingested cysts become trophozoites that invade the colon wall and cause a variety of intestinal symptoms.

Clinical Presentation

Most individuals are asymptomatic, and many become chronic carriers.

Symptomatic individuals may develop alternating constipation and diarrhea over 1 to 3 weeks, abdominal cramping, weight loss, anorexia, and nausea.

More severe infections may develop weeks to months after infection, resulting in symptoms of dysentery with fever and bloody stools.

Trophozoites may migrate to other locations in the body including the liver, skin, heart, and brain. Liver abscesses can form acutely or may develop years after infection with symptoms of fever, RUQ pain, and weight loss.

Treatment

- Empiric treatment for amebiasis may be initiated in a patient with dysentery who does not respond to an appropriate antibiotic.
- Diagnosis may be made by stool ova and parasite examination if the patient seeks medical treatment either during or after travel.

Cryptosporidium

Pathophysiology

- *Cryptosporidium* is a protozoan that is present throughout the environment, including up to 97% of large streams, lakes and reservoirs in the U.S. The organism is introduced to various water sources from the feces of infected animals.
- *Cryptosporidium* is resistant to iodine and chlorine disinfectants.
- Transmission may occur through ingestion of contaminated water and possibly food.

Clinical Presentation

- Cryptosporidia typically cause a self-limited diarrheal illness that develops 2 – 14 days after ingestion.
- Symptoms include watery diarrhea, crampy abdominal pain, anorexia, malaise, and flatulence.
- Severity of disease varies from asymptomatic infection to stools occurring more than seventy times daily in patients with poor immune systems.

Treatment

- No effective treatment has been found, and eradication of the infection is the result of the patient's own immune function.
- Supportive therapy consists of fluid and electrolyte replacement.

Other Gastrointestinal Infections

Hepatitis A

Pathophysiology

- Hepatitis A virus causes acute inflammation of the liver.
- It is transmitted fecal-orally through direct contact or through contaminated food or water.
- It is present worldwide but is more common in developing nations.
- Undercooked shellfish from contaminated water is the most common source of transmission.

Clinical Presentation

- Incubation period from the time of ingestion is 15 – 50 days.
- Symptoms vary from mild gastroenteritis to fulminant liver failure.

Typical presentation includes acute onset of fever, lethargy, anorexia, nausea followed by darkening of urine (usually after 3 – 10 days), and jaundice.

■ Abdominal pain and vomiting, as well as itching and joint pain, may be present.

Livers and spleens can get very large.

Symptoms usually resolve without treatment in several days to two weeks, with jaundice resolving after three to four weeks.

Chronic infection does not occur.

Liver failure is a rare complication

Treatment

Provide supportive care, and evacuate for advanced medical care if symptoms become severe.

No specific medical therapy is available.

Prevention

Hepatitis A vaccine is recommended for all travelers to developing nations. A single dose vaccine followed by a booster at 6-12 months provides protection for 10 years.

Unimmunized contacts of hepatitis A patients should receive an injection of gamma globulin 0.2 ml/kg.

Appropriate measures for hygiene and water disinfection should be followed vigilantly.

Typhoid fever

Pathophysiology

Typhoid fever is a systemic illness caused primarily by the organism *Salmonella typhi*.

Typhoid fever occurs worldwide but is most commonly contracted in developing nations.

Humans are the only hosts for *S. typhi* and transmission occurs most commonly through ingestion of contaminated food and water.

Contact with chronic carriers of *S. typhi* may also lead to infection.

Once ingested, the bacteria penetrate the intestinal mucosa, causing bacterial enteritis as well as bacteremia and systemic illness.

Clinical Presentation

The incubation period of *S. typhi* is seven to fourteen days.

Initial symptoms include fever, headache, abdominal pain and malaise.

Gastroenteritis may occur early in the disease but often does not present during the first ten days of illness. Constipation may also occur.

The temperature rises slowly during the first week of the disease. During weeks two and three, a continuous high fever up to 104° F (40° C) persists.

A notable feature of the fever is a slowing of the heart rate.

A characteristic rash of "rose spots," 2 – 4 mm round flat blanching lesions, may appear on the trunk during days 7-10 of the illness.

Physical exam may reveal splenomegaly after the first week.

- Worsening diarrhea may develop during the third week.
- After three weeks, the fever typically begins to go away and symptoms begin to resolve spontaneously in uncomplicated cases.
- Complications of typhoid fever include intestinal perforation, gastrointestinal hemorrhage, sepsis with multi-system failure, and pneumonia.

Treatment

- Treatment of typhoid fever involves supportive care and management of fluids and electrolytes.
- Antibiotic treatment reduces the duration of disease and decreases the complication rate.

Prevention of Gastrointestinal Disease

- Proper hygiene and sanitation practices are essential in preventing infectious diseases of the GI tract.
- The wilderness traveler must be vigilant to ensure that food and water do not become contaminated.
- Wash hands thoroughly with soap or hand disinfectant before preparing and eating meals.
- Cooking and eating utensils should be cleaned with boiling water or bleach solution prior to each use.
- Diet
  - ☐ Avoid raw or undercooked meat, fish and seafood.
  - ☐ When traveling internationally, avoid street vendors, raw vegetables, and fresh salads.
  - ☐ Avoid unpasteurized milk, cheese, and other dairy products.
  - ☐ Peeled fruits and vegetables are generally safe.
  - ☐ Do not rinse food in water that has not been disinfected.
- Water
  - ☐ Use appropriate methods of water disinfection.
  - ☐ When traveling internationally, avoid tap water and ice cubes made from untreated water.
  - ☐ Purchase name brand bottled water.
    - It is important that you always check the seal on any water bottle prior to drinking; if dining out, request that you break the seal and open the bottle yourself.
    - Sometimes the vendors will recycle the bottles and fill them with tap water. Of course, they will bring the open water bottle to your table so that you will not recognize this trick.
- Prophylaxis
  - ☐ Bismuth subsalicylate has been shown to be safe and effective in preventing of diarrheal illness, reducing incidence of disease by up to 65%.
    - The recommended regimen is 2 tablets or 2 tablespoons four times daily.
    - Side effects include darkened stools and tongue and possibly constipation and nausea.
  - ☐ Avoid concurrent aspirin use.
  - ☐ In general, antibiotic prophylaxis is not recommended.
  - ☐ In short-term trips to high-risk areas where circumstances may demand more aggressive strategies of prevention, usually use broad-spectrum antibiotics.

Evacuation Guidelines

- Any victim with moderate to severe abdominal pain that does not improve over 12 – 24 hours should be evacuated.
- Victims unable to tolerate sufficient oral rehydration fluids for more than 24 hours should be evacuated.

- Anyone experiencing mental status changes, signs of significant dehydration, hematemesis, or copious bloody stools should be evacuated immediately.
- Victims with signs and symptoms of dysentery who do not respond to appropriate antibiotic therapy in 24 – 48 hours should be evacuated.

MALARIA

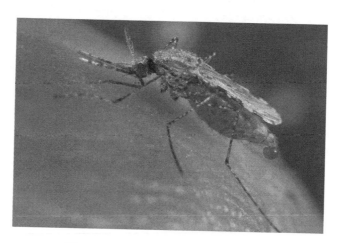

Figure 17.1 Anopheles Mosquito

Pathophysiology

- Malaria is a parasitic infection caused by protozoa of the genus *Plasmodium*.
- Malaria is one the most common infections worldwide, with 300 – 500 million cases occurring annually with over 2.5 million deaths.
- The female *Anopheles* mosquito transmits the parasites, which invade and destroy red blood cells.
- They typically bite at nights

Four species of Plasmodium cause malaria

Organism	Distribution
Plasmodium falciparum	Worldwide, esp. sub-Saharan Africa, Amazon, Haiti, SE Asia
Plasmodium vivax	Worldwide, esp. Mexico, Central America, N. Africa, Middle East, India
Plasmodium ovale	West Africa
Plasmodium malariae	Worldwide

Clinical presentation

- Symptoms typically present one to two weeks after exposure to an infected mosquito.
- Initial symptoms include muscle soreness and low-grade fever, which progress to paroxysms of shaking chills followed by high-grade fever and drenching sweats.
- Cycles of chills and fever last several hours and may occur every two to three days, depending on the specific organism.
- Headaches, muscles aches, and backaches are also common and may be severe.
- Other symptoms include nausea, vomiting, diarrhea, severe anemia, and darkened urine (aka blackwater fever).
- Severe *P. falciparum* infection may present with constant fever and high levels of parasites that can lead to cerebral malaria.
  - Symptoms of cerebral malaria include high fever, confusion, coma, seizures, and possibly death.
  - Mortality rates of cerebral malaria are greater than 20%.
  - Other complications of severe infection include pulmonary edema, acute renal failure, profound hypoglycemia, and lactic acidosis.

Prevention

- A combination of personal protective measures and medicines is essential to avoid malaria infection in endemic areas.
- The *Anopheles* mosquito is most likely to bite between dusk and dawn.
  - Limit exposure by using mosquito nets and wearing protective clothing impregnated with an insecticide such as Permethrin.
  - Light-colored clothes with long sleeves and long pants are recommended.
  - Insect repellent containing DEET (no higher than 35% concentration is necessary) should be applied to exposed skin.
- Consult with a travel clinic or review the CDC recommendations to determine the appropriate chemoprophylaxis for the region of travel (http://www.cdc.gov/travel).

Treatment

- Malaria infection can occur despite careful behavior modification and chemoprophylaxis. For wilderness travel in endemic areas, appropriate medications should be taken for self treatment.
- Recommended treatment regimens should be determined through consultation with a travel clinic or the CDC.
- Treatment should be initiated when signs and symptoms suggest malarial infection and medical care is not immediately available.
- Anyone suspected of having malaria should be evacuated, especially in areas where *P. falciparum* is predominant.

RABIES

Pathophysiology

- Rabies is caused by a virus.
- The virus is transmitted in the saliva of infected animals.
- Only two to three deaths are reported annually in the U.S., but worldwide an estimated 55,000 people die each year from rabies.
- In the U.S., over 90% of animal rabies occurs in wildlife, with less than 5% occurring in dogs.
- In most developing nations, however, dogs account for up to 90% of reported animal rabies.
- Major vectors for rabies worldwide include dogs, bats, foxes, raccoons, skunks, coyotes, and mongooses. Bats are the most common vector for human infection in the U.S. unlikely animal vectors include small rodents, birds, and reptiles.
- Worldwide, dogs remain the biggest threat for the transmission or rabies.
- Following inoculation, the rabies virus travels through the peripheral nervous system to the central nervous system. The virus multiplies in the central nervous system and then spreads throughout the body via the cranial and peripheral nerves.

Treatment

- There is no proven therapy for treatment of rabies.
- Anyone suspected of exposure should undergo appropriate post-exposure prophylaxis.
- In the USA the Centers for Disease Control (CDC) has a number for advice for people who have received a bite. (888) 232-6348 http://www.cdc.gov/travel

Prevention

- Wilderness travelers most at risk include spelunkers, professional hunters, wildlife workers, and those traveling to endemic areas for extended periods or to remote areas without medical care.
- If someone has received a bite it is important to wash the wound.

TICK-BORNE DISEASES

Lyme Disease

Pathophysiology

- Lyme disease is caused by the spirochete *Borrelia burgdorferi*.
- It is transmitted by *Ixodes* species ticks.
- 12 U.S. states report 95% of cases: Massachusetts, Connecticut, Maine, New Hampshire, Rhode Island, New York, New Jersey, Pennsylvania, Delaware, Maryland, Michigan, and Wisconsin.

Clinical Presentation

Lyme disease presents with three distinct stages.

Stage I
- Usually develops three days to one month after a tick bite.
- 55% of patients develop the classic rash called *erythema chronicum migrans*. This is a characteristic rash that may be uniformly red or have a more complex "bull's eye" appearance due to central clearing.
- Other symptoms
  * Malaise, fatigue, lethargy   80%
  * Headache   64%
  * Fever and chills   59%
  * Stiff neck   48%
  * Multiple annular lesions   48%
  * Regional lymphadenopathy   41%

Stage II: early disseminated infection
- Includes neurologic problems, such as meningitis, cranial nerve palsies Cardiac problems, such as heart inflammation and heart block, may also be present.

Stage III: late disseminated disease due to partially or untreated infection
- Occurs months to years later with arthritis, often involving the knee.
- Chronic neurologic complications can occur including pain, vertigo, weakness, and cognitive impairments.

Treatment

Antibiotics

Rocky Mountain Spotted Fever

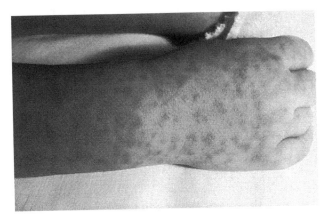

Figure 17.2 Rocky Mountain Spotted Fever

Pathophysiology

RMSF is a serious disease caused by the spirochete *Rickettsia rickettsii*.

The spirochete is transmitted by the Ixodes ticks

Despite its name, most cases occur in southern and eastern states of the U.S.

Reported mortality rates range from 3% – 9%.

Clinical Presentation

- Most cases present during spring and early summer, but infections can occur throughout the year.
- The incubation time is 12 – 14 days.
- Early symptoms may be nonspecific and include mild chills, anorexia, and malaise, which then progress to the classic triad of fever, severe headache, and rash. Other symptoms include muscle aches, bone pain, abdominal pain, and confusion.
- The rash characteristically begins on the extremities and spreads to the trunk. It includes the palms and soles. The rash starts as a round, flat rash and progresses to a pin point rash. Patients may appear quite toxic and the majority requires hospitalization.

Treatment

- In addition to supportive care, antibiotics are also given
- Treatment should be continued for at least three days after the fever goes away.
- Any patient suspected of RMSF infection should be evacuated immediately.

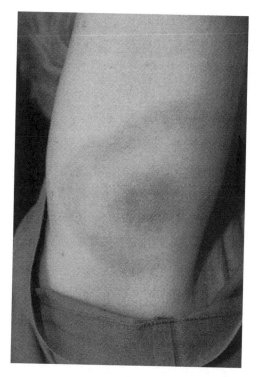

Figure 17.3. Lyme disease – Erythema Chronicum Migrans rash

Tick Paralysis

Pathophysiology

- Tick paralysis is an acute, ascending, muscle paralysis caused by neurotoxic venom secreted from the salivary glands of ticks.
- In the U.S., most cases occur in the Pacific Northwest and the Rocky Mountain areas.
- There is a similar tick paralysis in Australia that has greater death rate.
- April through June are the highest months of risk in the U.S.

Clinical Presentation

- Symptoms typically develop five to seven days after tick attachment.
- Early symptoms may include irritability and numbness of the hands and feet.
- Over 24 – 48 hours, ascending paralysis develops with loss of deep tendon reflexes.

Treatment

- Treatment involves removal of the tick and supportive care.
- Symptoms usually resolve within hours to one day after removal.
- In Australia, there is an antivenin to administer before removal of the tick. The antivenin is given because victims usually worsen after removal of the tick.

Colorado Tick Fever

Pathophysiology

- Colorado tick fever is a viral illness transmitted by the wood tick, primarily during spring and early summer.
- Most cases occur in mountainous regions of the Western U.S. and Canada.

Clinical Presentation

- The average incubation time is three to four days.
- Symptoms include fever, chills, lethargy, headache, muscle aches, eye pain, photophobia, abdominal pain, nausea, and vomiting.
- A rash occurs in 5% – 12% of infected patients.
- Acute symptoms last up to one week, with fatigue sometimes lasting much longer.
- 5% – 10% of children develop meningitis or encephalitis.

Treatment

- Treatment is supportive.
- Persons with symptoms of Colorado tick fever should be evacuated for medical evaluation.

QUESTIONS

1. While traveling abroad in Guatemala, you and a friend run out of water when spending several days backpacking in the mountains. You decide to drink from a local stream to quench your thirst. Several hours later both you and your friend begin to have abdominal cramps with copious amounts of watery diarrhea that looks like rice water. What is the appropriate treatment for your condition?
   a) Extensive antibiotic therapy along with vaccine
   b) Nothing, the symptoms will wear off in a few hours
   c) Drink Gatorade and other electrolyte containing drinks to counteract effects of water loss
   d) Sugar pills

2. Your brother returns from a trip to Connecticut, USA where he went camping in the woods for a few days. He soon develops a fever, headache, and a rash that begins on his wrists and ankles then spreads to his palms and soles. The rash is characterized by central clearing. How did your friend contract this illness?
   a) A tick bite
   b) A mosquito bite
   c) Poor water sanitation
   d) Close contact with a rabid animal

3. Your younger brother goes swimming in a local chlorinated pool here in Utah and develops abdominal pain and watery diarrhea three days later. What organism is most likely responsible for his symptoms?
   a) Giardia lamblia
   b) Shigella species
   c) Salmonella
   d) Cryptosporidium

4. With regards to the previous question, what is the proper treatment of your younger brother's illness?
   a) IV antibiotic therapy
   b) Anti-toxin
   c) Vaccination
   d) The virus is self-limited and the body's immune system can take care of it

5. **While hiking in the backcountry you come across a person who was bitten by a rabid raccoon. The person states that they are afraid that the raccoon had rabies because "it had white stuff coming out of its mouth." What should you advise the person to do?**
   a) Nothing, once you are inoculated with rabies you are a dead man. Tell the person not to feed wild animals in the afterlife.
   b) Quickly find the nearest hospital to receive post-exposure prophylaxis
   c) Use a knife to cut off the bite
   d) Sufficient water plus over-the-counter pain medication

ANSWERS
1.c 2. a 3. d 4. d 5. b

CHAPTER 18

Law and the Wilderness

Case

A backpacker trained in basic life support and wilderness emergency care comes across a group of people surrounding a collapsed man. The man is lying with his back on the ground and is holding his head. The backpacker inquires as to the status of the man but never identifies himself as being trained in life support. The people surrounding the man said that he fell while trying to climb a nearby tree to take a picture of the group. The backpacker decides to continue on his way back down the trail because the fallen man doesn't appear to be in an emergency situation, and he wants to make it back to his car before sundown because his flashlight has run out of battery.

■ What is the backpacker's responsibility?
■ What might happen to the backpacker if the fallen man had a severe head injury, such as a hematoma, that could cause death?

LEGAL CONCERNS IN THE WILDERNESS

The welfare of the people is the ultimate law – Cicero

- When encountering an accident victim or a person experiencing some other medical emergency in the backcountry, a person's instinct is to provide medical care.
- The most important aspect of treating a patient in the back country is assuring skilled, efficient care
- Concerns about legal liability should be a very distant, tertiary factor.
- Nonetheless, because of an increasingly litigious world, concerns about legal liability could intrude upon the caregiver.
- Those liability concerns, however, can be eliminated or at least reduced by understanding and then conforming one's behavior to a few legal principles.

consent is often assumed

GOOD SAMARITAN LAWS — *to encourage people to provide care*

Affirmative Obligation to Help

will not cover neglect i.e. you caused injury b/c you gave up, you were paid

In the United States, the most extreme reactions to this common law rule are found in Minnesota, Rhode Island and Vermont, where each has enacted a statute requiring a person to render aid, under certain conditions, to a stranger found in an emergency situation.

The Minnesota statute, quoted in part below, is a good example of this type of legislation:

> *A person at. . .an emergency who knows that another person is exposed to or has suffered grave physical harm shall, to the extent that the person can do so without danger. . .to self or others, give reasonable assistance to the exposed person. . . .*

- The Province of Quebec in Canada and virtually every country on the European Continent have similar statutory requirements.
- Therefore, when traveling in the backcountry in Europe, Quebec, Minnesota, Rhode Island, and Vermont, remember that you are obligated to give reasonable aid and assistance to a stranger suffering or exposed to grave physical harm or otherwise found in an emergency situation.
- Depending on the circumstances and the particular jurisdiction's law, your obligation to help might be satisfied by immediately reporting the situation to the proper authorities that can provide help and aid to the victim.
- Most jurisdictions that impose this obligation to render emergency care generally also have a limitation of liability statute as described below.

Limitation of Liability

- Some U.S. States have laws to encourage people to aid others in emergencies by limiting liability.
- All of the U.S. states and many other common law jurisdictions (in Canada, Alberta, British Colombia, Nova Scotia, and Ontario) have enacted Good Samaritan laws.
- Good Samaritan under certain circumstances, protect a person who voluntarily renders emergency care.
- Although these statutes differ in language among jurisdictions, all are very similar in purpose, rest upon the same fundamental principles, and have the same requirements.

■ The Utah statute (USA) quoted below is a good example of these laws:

A person who renders emergency care at or near the scene of, or during an emergency, gratuitously and on good faith, is not liable for any civil damages or penalties as a result of any act or omission by the person rendering the emergency care, unless the person is grossly negligent or caused the emergency.

■ In any jurisdiction, for the Good Samaritan law to apply and protect a person rendering emergency care, the following five general principles must be scrupulously observed:

1. **The person rendering emergency care must not have caused the emergency either in whole or in part.**

2. **The person rendering emergency care must act in "good faith."** The care provider must sincerely intend to help and must have a reasonable opinion that the care should not be postponed until the patient is hospitalized.

3. **The emergency care must be provided without any compensation.** The care provider should not accept anything in return for rendering the emergency care.

4. **The provider must not commit gross negligence when rendering emergency care.** To list all possible acts that might constitute gross negligence is impossible. The best practice is simply to provide emergency care in accordance with the accepted medical standards. Be advised that once initiating emergency aid in the back country and then either terminating treatment or transferring care of the patient to an inadequately trained person before the patient is adequately stabilized or evacuated to a medical facility can be considered abandonment, which is gross negligence.

5. **The person rendering emergency care must not have a preexisting duty to care for the patient.** For example, a guide would have a preexisting duty to render emergency care to a customer where that customer had contracted with the guide to be taken on a hike and the guide had agreed to provide care to the customer in case of injury while hiking.

Contract Law

A contract is an agreement, or a promise, between two or more parties for performing certain specified acts in exchange for adequate compensation.

Contracts can be either "expressed" or "implied."

The terms of an express contract are explicitly stated in words, either written or oral, leaving little or no doubt as to its existence and terms.

An implied contract is not expressly set forth, either orally or in writing.

Rather, the existence and terms of an implied contract are created by conduct or circumstances that "imply" a contract exist.

Contracts, letter agreements, or even brochures from summer camps, expedition companies and adventure guides sometimes expressly state they have a trained person available to provide medical care to customers in emergencies arising during the adventure activity.

Alternatively, the oral sales presentation or even the brochure may well "imply" that the summer camp, expedition company, or adventure guide will provide such medical aid to customers under its care.

In either situation, express or implied, a court may find that the complaining customer stayed at the camp or took the adventurous expedition in part because the company or guide contractually agreed to provide medical aid during back country emergencies.

This created a preexisting duty on the part of the company or guide that renders the Good Samaritan law inapplicable.

The complaining patient can sue the provider of backcountry emergency medical aid for ordinary negligence and perhaps recover money damages.

With the Good Samaritan law out of the way, that lawsuit would proceed under tort law.

Tort Law

Tort law sets civil standards for people's behavior, imposing on everyone the duty to exercise reasonable care to avoid causing harm or injury to others and providing legal recourse and the possible recovery of money damages for those who suffer harm or injury as a result of a breach of this duty.

Torts are legally defined civil wrongs that might result in harm or injury and thereby constitute the basis for a claim (or law suit) by the harmed or injured party against the person who allegedly committed the tort.

An injured party can claim under any of three general categories of torts:

- (1) an intentional tort where one person intentionally harms or injures another
- (2) a strict liability tort such as making and selling an obviously defective product
- (3) a negligent tort where a careless and unintentional act, such as an automobile accident

Among harms or injuries suffered by a party for which it could recover a monetary award in tort litigation are compensation for:

- (1) lost income and lost or damaged property
- (2) pain and suffering
- (3) reasonable medical expenses.

Four Elements of a Negligence Claim

In order to prove that a person (the defendant) who provided emergency medical care in the backcountry committed a tort of negligence, the person who claims to have been harmed or injured by that emergency medical care (the plaintiff) must prove the following four elements of a negligence claim:

Duty to Provide Care at the Standard of Care

- The plaintiff must demonstrate that the defendant had a duty to provide aid to the plaintiff that met a specified standard of care.
- Although training courses such as this are making great progress in defining and refining the standard of care in wilderness medicine, that standard is not yet well established in the law. When in doubt, courts will rely upon the traditional legal definition of the standard of care, which is the "behavior of a reasonably prudent person in the same or similar circumstances."
- In applying the traditional legal definition, courts commonly look to the following factors to determine the applicable standard of care:
  1. The defendant's education
  2. The defendant's training
  3. Government or organization medical protocols that apply to the particular situation
  4. Industry practice
  5. Private business protocols that might apply

Failure to Perform the Duty

- The plaintiff must next prove the defendant failed to perform the duty of providing aid consistent with the specified standard of care.
- This proof can take several forms. In most wilderness medicine litigations, the plaintiff asserts the defendant failed to act at all (an omission) when the defendant had a preexisting duty to provide care to the plaintiff.

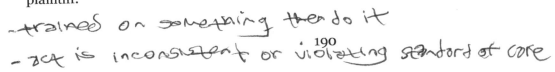

(handwritten) —trained on something then do it
(handwritten) —act is inconsistent or violating standard of care

190

- ○ The plaintiff might, however, claim the defendant provided care (a commission) that did not meet the prevailing medical standard or did not perform as would a reasonable person with the defendant's background, education, and training.
- ○ The premature termination of care or the transfer of care to a less-qualified provider before the patient has been stabilized or evacuated can, as mentioned above, be considered abandonment and constitute negligence or even gross negligence.
- ○ Consequently, one must remain well informed of prevailing medical standards and protocols and be well trained in wilderness medicine to ensure that any care provided meets applicable standards.
- ■ **Loss or Injury**
  - ○ The plaintiff must next demonstrate that he or she sustained a loss or injury, which can include loss or damage to property, medical expenses, fright, emotional trauma, personal injury, pain and suffering, or loss of life.

- ■ **Causation**
  - ○ Finally, the plaintiff must demonstrate that the loss or injury sustained was caused or contributed to (the "proximate cause") by the defendant's failure to perform the duty of providing aid meeting the specified standard of care.

Defenses to a Tort Law Claim

- ■ The defendant can defeat the plaintiff's claim by demonstrating that the plaintiff failed to carry the burden of proof on one or more of the four elements of a negligence claim.
- ■ For example, the defendant might demonstrate that he or she satisfied the duty of performing in accordance with the applicable standard of care or another person or event caused that the plaintiff's loss or injury.
- ■ The best strategy always is to keep a contemporaneous, complete, and accurate written record of the events surrounding and the medical care given in response to a back country or wilderness emergency.
- ■ Such records should include dates and times, a patient history, a description of the scene, your physical assessment, treatment given, and any changes in the patient while in your care.
- ■ Experience teaches that such a record is an essential element in any successful defense.

Standard of care:
- depends on - education, training, gov't protocol, industry practice, private business protocols
Doctor is charge - always makes the call

Documentation - this is important!
(esp. if you leave them or they don't take your advice

QUESTIONS

1. In the state of Utah in the USA, which one of the following is NOT a general principle of the Good Samaritan Laws?
   a) The person rendering emergency care must not have caused the emergency
   b) The person providing care must receive written permission from the injured in order to provide care
   c) The provider must not commit gross negligence when rendering emergency care
   d) The emergency care must be provided gratuitously, without any compensation

2. In applying the traditional legal definition, which one of the following do the courts look to in order to determine the applicable standard of care in a negligence case?
   a) The defendant's training
   b) The defendant's racial background
   c) The defendant's alcohol level at the time
   d) The weather in which the defendant was exposed when assisting the injured

3. What are torts?
   a) Common law of the backcountry land specific to a wilderness area
   b) Original Native American humanitarian laws that have been applied treating people in the backcountry
   c) Legally defined civil wrongs that might result in harm or injury and, thereby, constitute the basis for a claim
   d) Important procedures used to define healthcare in the wilderness

4. Which of the following is a necessary element in a negligence claim?
   a) Causation
   b) Financial standing of the care provider
   c) Sufficient concern towards the comfort level of the person receiving care
   d) Land terrain where the accident occurred

ANSWERS
1. b 2. a 3. c 4. a

CHAPTER 19

Lightning Injuries and Prevention

This chapter will train you to recognize and treat injuries caused by lightning strikes and ways to avoid being struck by lightning.

Objectives:

- Recognize when and where lightning is more likely to strike in relation to a storm
- Be able to describe the six mechanisms by which one may be struck by lightning
- Understand the concept of "reverse triage" in managing multiple casualties from a lightning strike
- Understand that all victims of a lightning strike should be evacuated as soon as possible from the wilderness
- Be able to list several methods to minimize the potential that one may be struck by lightning while in the wilderness

Case

A 23-year-old male is leaning against a vehicle when the large whip antenna is stuck by lightning. He is thrown back from the vehicle and is slightly confused about what actually happened. On your evaluation, he is awake and alert. He remembers a large flash of light. The next thing he remembers is being on the ground 10 feet away from the vehicle. His physical examination is normal, with the exception of an unusual rash on his left chest (pictured below).

1. What is the next step in the management of this victim?
2. Are you at risk of electrical injury from a residual electrical charge if you touch him?
3. Does he require evacuation to a hospital, or can he stay in the wilderness and continue his journey.

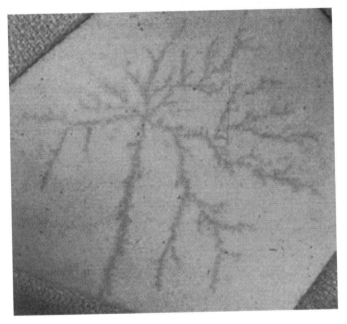

Figure 19.1 Rash on the Left Side of the Chest of the Case

TYPES OF LIGHTNING INJURIES

Direct strike

- The victim is struck directly by the bolt of lightning.
- This most commonly occurs to people who are caught in the open and are unable to find cover.

Side splash

- The lightning directly strikes another object such as a tree or building, but the current flow, which seeks the path of least resistance, jumps from its original pathway onto the victim.
- This is the most common cause of lightning injury.
- Side splashes may also splash indoors from metal objects, such as plumbing and telephones.
- Splashes may occur from person to person when several people are standing close together.

Contact

- Contact exposure occurs when a person is holding onto or touching an object that is either directly hit or splashed by lightning.
- The current passes through the object to the victim.

Ground current or step voltage

- Ground current is produced when lightning strikes the ground or a nearby object and the current spreads through the ground.
- If a person has one foot closer to the strike, then a potential difference may exist between the two feet and the current will pass up one leg and down the other leg.
- This occurs because the body is of lower resistance than the ground.
- This is a common mechanism for several people being injured at the same time.

Injury by a weak upward streamer

- The electrical streamer heads upward into the sky but does not reach sky lightning, thus not completing a connection.
- The electrical charge passes over and through the involved individual but at a lesser energy than the amount from a direct strike from the sky.

Blunt trauma

- The injury occurs due to the impact of the concussive force of the strike itself, or due to being thrown because of the extreme nature of muscular contractions from the electrical charge.

INJURIES CAUSED BY LIGHTNING

Heart

- The most common cause of death in a lightning victim is cardiopulmonary arrest from an abnormal heart rhythm.
- A victim may suffer an initial cardiac arrest but recover his heartbeat in a period of seconds to minutes. However, if the victim sustains concomitant respiratory arrest due to inactivity of the respiratory drive center,

which is very common, he may sustain a second cardiac arrest due to lack of oxygen from not breathing. The drive to breathe usually occurs later than when the heart starts beating on its own. That is why it is important to anticipate the need to continue rescue breathing for victims even if they recover a pulse.

Central nervous system

- Bleeding in the brain can occur from a current that traverses the brain.
- Victims who sustain burns to the head are four times more likely to die than those without cranial burns.
- Seizures may occur after a lightning strike.
- Confusion and amnesia are very common.
- Long-term effects may include memory impairment, difficulty concentrating, sleep disturbances, and personality changes.
- Temporary paralysis of the upper or lower extremities can occur.

Respiratory system

- The victim may stop breathing from the lightning strike due to injury-induced malfunction of their respiratory drive center.
- The victim may sustain contusions (bruises) to the lung and cough up bloody sputum.

Skin

- Contrary to popular myth and what is seen in cartoons, deep burns are unusual after lightning injury. At the most, some minor partial thickness burns may occur from superheated metal objects in contact with the skin.
- Often there are no burns, especially with ground current.
- There are four types of common skin effects:
  o Ferning (see image from the case): Also called feathering or Lichtenberg figures. These are not actual burns, but an unusual pattern that occurs due to the electron shower that courses over the skin surface.
  o Linear burns: These are usually first and second degree burns that occur from steam production from sweat or water that instantaneously heats and evaporates on the victim due to the increased temperatures associated with the lightning strike.
  o Punctate burns: These are multiple, closely spaced, but discrete circular burns that individually range from a few millimeters to a centimeter in thickness.
  o Thermal burns: These are regular thermal burns that occur when a victim is wearing a metal object, such as a belt buckle or necklace, which heats up due to the electrical current traversing it. There may also be thermal burns if clothing ignites.

Musculoskeletal system

- Fractures and dislocations may occur due to intense muscular contractions or from the trauma of being thrown.

Ear

- Temporary deafness can occur due to the intense noise and shock wave.
- 30% to 50% of victims rupture one or both ear drums.
- Victims who were using a conventional (wired) telephone at the time of the strike are at high risk for hearing injuries, especially if there is a side splash into a dwelling through the telephone.

Eye

- Temporary blindness of both eyes may occur, but this is usually temporary
- Cataracts are very common and may occur immediately or more commonly weeks to months later.
- Multiple types of internal eye damage can occur.
- Fixed dilated pupils occur as well, so do not rely on this as an absolute sign of death in a victim of lightning strike.

SIGNS OF LIGHTNING INJURY

Single Victim

- Identification of a victim of a lightning strike is readily made if the strike was witnessed.
- In the case of the unwitnessed strike victim, clues that can assist you include environmental conditions, such as a recent thunderstorm or lightning.
- If the victim displays confusion and amnesia, as well as prominent physical findings such as ruptured ear drums and the classic skin finding of ferning, these findings assist in the diagnosis.

Multiple Victims

- The typical description of a multiple casualty lightning strike is one of a sudden flash of bright light followed closely by a loud boom and then chaos.
- There will likely be several people who are walking around but are confused. There will be people who are lying on the ground but are moving or breathing on their own. These first two groups of people do not require immediate attention.
- The final group of casualties may include one to several people who are unconscious, not breathing, and do not have a pulse. This final group is the one that requires immediate attention. The fact that you are first treating persons who appear dead is called "reverse triage." The reason for this reverse triage is due to the fact that victims who are awake or breathing have survived the most immediate and potentially critical injury, which is cardiac and respiratory arrest.
- Victims who are not breathing and have no pulse require CPR. Some of these victims will regain a heartbeat and respiratory drive, but it may take up to 10-15 minutes before this occurs. Performing CPR on these victims can save their lives if their heart and brain are not too severely damaged.
- In attempting to decide on which victims you should start the CPR, remember that those with head burns are four times more likely to die than persons without head burns.

TREATMENT OF LIGHTNING INJURY

- Perform reverse triage and initiate CPR on victims who are not breathing and have no pulse before caring for those who have spontaneous signs of life.
- Victims without spontaneous breathing or heartbeat may recover their heartbeat and will require assisted breathing until their respiratory drive returns. Breathing for these victims may prevent secondary cardiac arrest due to lack of oxygen.
- Call for evacuation to the closest medical facility.
- Stabilization and splinting of fractures and dislocations and spinal precautions should be performed as determined by the secondary assessment.
- Lightning does not leave a residual electrical charge on a victim of a strike. There is no need to be concerned about getting shocked by rescuing a person who has been struck by lightning.

PREVENTION

The 30-30 rule

- The 1st "30": When the time between seeing a bolt of lightning and/or just hearing thunder is 30 seconds or less, then people are in danger and should be seeking appropriate cover.
- The 2nd "30": Outdoor activities should not be resumed until 30 minutes after the last lightning is seen or the last thunder heard.
- The worst times for a lightning strike are right before the storm hits and just after it passes. It is actually less dangerous during the storm, but one must still take full precautions.

Seek shelter in a substantial building or in an all-metal vehicle

- Small shelters, such as golf carts, buses, and rain shelters, may increase a person's risk of being struck due to side splash as the lightning flows over the shelter.
- All metal vehicles are safe because the metal will diffuse the current around the occupants to the ground. A convertible automobile is not a safe alternative. It is a myth that the rubber tires on a vehicle provide insulation.

If you are caught in a storm outside without a safe building or vehicle

- Stay away from metal objects and items that are taller than you.
- Avoid areas near power lines, pipelines, ski lifts, and other large steel objects.
- Do not stand near or under tall isolated trees, hilltops, or at a lookout or other exposed area.
- In a forest, seek a low area under a growth of saplings or small trees. Seeking a clearing free of trees makes a person the tallest object in the clearing.
- If you are in a group of people, spread far apart so that a single lightning strike will not take out the entire group.
- If on the water, seek the shore and avoid being the tallest object near a large body of water.
- The more dangerous times for a severe lightning strike are before the storm appears and after it has passed.

- Lightning does strike twice in the same place - all the time.
- If you are totally in the open, stay far away from single trees to avoid lightning splashes and ground current. A good position is to squat down with your knees fully bent and your feet together. This way a current will go through your feet and not through your heart. You can also sit cross-legged if you want. Try to cover your ears so that thunder will not damage your hearing.

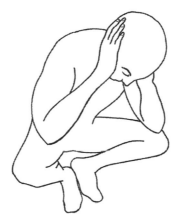

Figure 19.2 Lightning Position

If indoors

- Avoid open doors and windows, fireplaces, and metal objects, such as sinks, and plug in electrical appliances.
- Do not talk on the telephone (even a cordless phone), because telephone lines are usually not grounded in the same method as electrical wires.

EVACUATION GUIDELINES

- Any victim of a lightning strike should be evacuated as soon as possible.
- Even if the individual does not have any overt evidence of physical injury, there is a high likelihood of some sort of injury that is not served best by staying in the wilderness.

QUESTIONS

1. **What is the most dangerous time to be struck by lightning in relation to the storm?**
   a) The very first time you hear thunder
   b) In the middle of the storm, when the rain is hardest
   c) The period of time right before the storm actually hits
   d) Thirty-five minutes after the storm ends
   e) You are at the same risk regardless of the stage of the storm

2. **In which one of the following situations is somebody least likely to get injured by lightning?**
   a) Crouching near the top of a ridge line
   b) Sitting inside a rain shelter that is open from the front on a golf course
   c) Sitting under a large tree that provides protection from the rain
   d) Sitting in an all-metal automobile with the windows rolled up
   e) Standing upright in the middle of an open field

3. **A 30-year-old male is struck by lightning and is not breathing. Which one of the following is correct in regards to the management of this victim?**
   a) CPR is not necessary as his heart will resume beating on its own
   b) CPR is not helpful as his heart likely sustained irreversible damage
   c) CPR should be initiated until he begins breathing on his own, then you may stop
   d) CPR should be initiated until he regains his pulse, then you may stop
   e) CPR should not be initiated, because the victim may carry a residual charge from the lightning and thereby injure the rescuer

4. **You observe lightning strike a large group of people with the following casualties:**
   a) Awake, alert, and sitting up with obvious dislocated shoulder
   b) Awake, moaning, and confused
   c) Unconscious, not breathing, no evidence of injury
   d) Unconscious, not breathing, obvious burn to the head and face
   e) Unconscious, breathing on own

5. **What is the correct order that you should care for these victims?**
   a) A, B, E, D, C
   b) B, E, D, C, A
   c) C, D, E, B, A
   d) D, C, E, B, A
   e) E, C, D, B, A

6. Which one of the following is a method to minimize being struck by lightning?
   a) If caught in the open, squat down with your feet together
   b) Seek shelter under the largest tree out in the open, ensuring you are leaning against it
   c) Lay supine if you are caught in the open
   d) Seek shelter when you see lightning and hear thunder within 10 seconds
   e) Sit under large electrical towers because they are grounded and protected from lightning

ANSWERS

1. c   2. d   3. c   4. c   5. c

CHAPTER 20

Medical Problems in the Backcountry

This chapter will train you on how to recognize and evaluate common medical conditions while in the backcountry. It will help you to differentiate serious problems that require evacuation from minor problems that can be treated without evacuation.

Objectives:

- Evaluate and determine the need for evacuation of patients with chest pain in the backcountry.
- Evaluate and determine the need for evacuation of patients with shortness of breath in the backcountry.
- Understand and treat neurological problems.
- Understand and treat diabetic issues.
- Recognize and treat allergic reactions.
- Evaluate abdominal pain and know when patients need to be evacuated from the backcountry.
- Describe various methods that may be used to prevent the most common infectious diseases in wilderness travel.

- Identify when a patient with an infectious disease must be evacuated from the wilderness.

CHEST PAIN RELATED EMERGENCIES

Case 1

A 56-year-old man is on day four of a seven-day rafting trip on river. He is paddling a raft through a calm stretch of water. He begins to experience chest pain that spreads to his left shoulder. The pain is significant enough that he has to pull over to the shore. He describes pressure in his chest as well.

1. What questions should you ask this patient?
2. What are some life-threatening causes of chest pain?
3. Does he require evacuation or can he stay on the trip?

Chest pain can occur for many different reasons. Pain related to the heart, lungs, stomach, bones and muscles of the chest wall can all cause chest pain. The primary goal of the wilderness medicine provider is to try and determine if the cause of the chest pain is life threatening, and thus requires evacuation. This can be very difficult, even for a physician in a hospital setting. In general, the wilderness medicine provider should always practice the "better safe than sorry" philosophy when it comes to evaluating chest pain.

Heart-Related Chest Pain

There are several conditions that can cause chest pain related to the heart. Infection, trauma, heart muscle inflammation, and heart attacks are all serious causes of chest pain. A patient is more likely to have chest pain related to a heart attack or other life-threatening condition if they have any of the following conditions:

Age > 50
Medical history of high blood pressure, diabetes, or high cholesterol
Previous history of heart problems
Uses tobacco of any kind
Significantly overweight

Always use the SAMPLE and OPQRST acronyms discussed in the patient assessment chapter when obtaining a medical history and characterizing the patient's pain. If a patient's cause of chest pain is related to the heart, they may complain of one or more of the following symptoms:

Onset with activity: often the pain will start with activity, where the heart is beating faster and using more oxygen.
Chest pain or pressure: this is often described as a squeezing or tightness, often with a clenched fist over the chest. The pain is usually in the center of the chest, but may radiate to the left arm, jaw, neck or back.

- Shortness of breath: especially with activity (even light activity).
- Nausea or vomiting: this is a frequent symptom if the patient and the heart are strained.
- Dizziness and sweating

Other Causes of Chest Pain

There are many other life-threatening causes of chest pain for which further description is beyond the scope of this text. In general, any of the following associated historical features and symptoms should make the wilderness medicine provider suspicious of a life-threatening cause of pain:

- History of blood clots in the legs or lungs
- Difficulty breathing with activity or at rest that is worse than the patient typically experiences
- Severe uncontrolled chest pain after several episodes of vomiting
- Associated fever, sweating or lightheadedness
- Severe tearing pain that spreads to the back

Treatment

- Rest is the key to reducing oxygen demand of the heart muscle. Sitting is better than lying down. Standing is the best position but may not be possible if the patient is too weak.
- If a patient has a history of heart-related chest pain and carries medications for a heart condition (such as nitroglycerin), they can take them as previously instructed by their physician.
- Increasing oxygen delivery to the heart muscle is important as well. Descending to a lower altitude and administration of oxygen if available will increase oxygen supply to the heart.
- Given time and rest, patients may be able to hike slowly downhill, but do not allow them to exert or climb uphill if pain is recurrent.
- If a patient has any concerning historical features or symptoms, they should be evacuated. During an evacuation the best way to the hospital is the fastest way to the hospital, even if the patient needs to walk.

The diagnosis of heart-related chest pain is very complex, especially without the help of x-rays, blood work, and electrocardiography. A patient can still be having a heart attack or other life-threatening condition, even if they do not have any of the risk factors or symptoms listed above. IF IN DOUBT, always err on the side of rapid evacuation to emergency medical treatment.

RESPIRATORY EMERGENCIES

Case 2

A 22-year-old female begins to have difficulty breathing while hiking on a trip in Nepal. She is an asthmatic and carries asthma medication with her. You are four walking days from any city.

1. What can this person do to help her own condition?
2. What are some ways to help improve her shortness of breath?
3. At what point should she be evacuated?

Shortness of Breath

Individuals can experience shortness of breath for many reasons in the backcountry, including asthma, hyperventilation, pulmonary embolism, allergic reactions, pneumonia, emphysema, and high altitude pulmonary edema. These causes can be difficult to distinguish from one another, especially in the wilderness. The primary goal of the wilderness medicine provider is not necessarily to determine the exact cause of a patient's shortness of breath, but more to give the patient some relief and determine whether or not the individual needs rapid evacuation. The following historical features and symptoms are concerning and are more likely to result in evacuation from the backcountry:

- History of emphysema or COPD (chronic obstructive pulmonary disease)
- Worsening shortness of breath with activity (worse than the individual typically has with activity)
- Signs of a respiratory infection such as fever, chills, and productive cough associated with the shortness of breath
- Chest pain associated with shortness of breath
- ■ Coughing up blood and shortness of breath
- Severe asthma attack not responding to the patient's previously prescribed medications

Treatment

- Place the victim in a position that makes breathing as easy as possible. Minimize the patient's activities/exertion.
- Have the individual use any medications they have been previously prescribed for the condition (i.e. inhalers for asthma, etc.).
- Descend from altitude if possible.
- Apply oxygen if available.
- If the symptoms do not resolve after a brief rest period, the patient should be evacuated.
- If the symptoms resolve, but then continue to recur despite multiple rest periods and treatment, the individual should be evacuated.
- Consider an infectious process such as pneumonia as the etiology of the symptoms.
- Consider antibiotics to treat respiratory pathogens if an infection seems present.

NEUROLOGIC EMERGENCIES

Case 3

While in camp, a 44-year-old female begins to have a seizure on day three of a nine-day trip to the Grand Canyon on the Colorado River. She has never had seizures before.

1. What are some features of a true seizure?
2. What should be done for this patient during the seizure?
3. Does she require evacuation?

[handwritten annotations: can be partial or generalized — one part of body / └ not necessarily / an emergency, needs to / └ full body involvement / be monitored]

Seizures

Seizures can occur from a primary seizure disorder or secondary to an injury or illness. Patients with known seizure disorders typically take medications to prevent them from occurring. A true generalized seizure typically has the following features:

- An aura prior to the seizure where the patient may describe a sick feeling, an odd taste or strange smell
- Generalized shaking of the entire body
- Loss of bowel or bladder control
- Inability to speak or consciously control seizure activity
- A period of confusion after the seizure, often lasting 30 minutes to an hour

A seizure in a person without a seizure disorder can occur for many reasons, including the following:

- Low blood sugar
- Head injury
- Infection of the brain or spinal cord
- Exposure to some type of toxic substance
- Stroke

[handwritten annotations: phases: / tonic — rigid posture / clonic — jerking — don't restrain / postictal — no memory, confusion / — time the phases, so a doc knows]

Treatment

The primary role of the wilderness medicine provider is to protect a patient while they are actively seizing. Methods to help prevent secondary injury in a patient having a seizure include the following:

- A seizure must run its course once it has begun. However, while the wilderness medicine provider can't stop the seizure, the patient must be prevented from hurting him/herself.
- If the patient begins to turn blue or appears to be choking, attempt to open the airway using the methods discussed in the patient assessment chapter.
- Do not try and hold a patient down or restrain them unless they are in immediate danger of hurting themselves, such as on a narrow trail bordered by a cliff.
- Move objects away from the patient and move the patient away from cliffs, water, or other hazards.
- A patient cannot swallow their tongue, so do not try to put anything into the mouth.

[handwritten annotations: Status epilepticus — / persistent seizure causes suffocation]

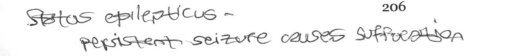

Once a patient stops seizing, they should be rolled onto their side (assuming they have not fallen a significant distance and there is no concern for neck injury) with their head supported by a pack or some folded clothing.

■ Check the patient from head to toe for injuries related to their seizure after they recover.

All first time seizures must be evacuated.

In the victim has a history of seizures, evacuation should be discussed with the person and a medical professional if at all possible.

If the seizure fails to stop or continues to recur for 30 minutes, the patient is considered to be in "status epilepticus" and will likely not stop without some type of intervention. DO NOT wait this long to arrange immediate evacuation from the wilderness. This is a true emergency because prolonged or recurrent seizures prevent adequate breathing and can lead to permanent injury.

In a person with a known seizure disorder, it is recommended that they be seizure free for at least six months before entering the backcountry. Another group member should always carry an extra set of the individual's anti-seizure medicines in case of loss or ruin of the primary set.

Cerebrovascular accident

Stroke

A stroke is an injury to an area of the brain, usually from lack of blood flow. Signs and symptoms vary depending on the part of the brain that is affected. A stroke may lead to one or more of the following symptoms:

Alteration in mental status (confusion, stupor, semi-consciousness, unconsciousness)

Decrease in muscle strength – usually on one side

Unsteady gait

Numbness – usually on one side

One-sided facial paralysis or facial drooping *weakness on one side*

Loss of reaction of one pupil to light *or numbness, tingling*

Blurred vision

Incontinence

- slowing & strong pulse

If one of these signs or symptoms occurs and then resolves within an hour, it is considered a transient ischemic attack (TIA), or a mini-stroke.

Treatment *- Evacuation, keep them calm - stay calm b/c they are cognating*

Strokes and TIA's can be severely debilitating and possibly life threatening. There is not much that can – or should – be done in the backcountry. *leave them in recovery position*

Make the patient as comfortable as possible. Patients who are unable to assume a comfortable position should be placed on the weak or paralyzed side to protect their airway.

Splint any paralyzed extremity to prevent it from being injured.

Evacuate as soon as possible.

Bells palsy
- similar, but can usually talk better

Bleeding stroke
- blood spilling out of vessel. leaves part of brain not getting blood

Clotting stroke
- blood unable to clot stroke

DIABETIC EMERGENCIES

Case 4

While hiking in the backcountry with a number of scouts, you are called to examine a 14-year-old boy who is becoming unresponsive. He is a known diabetic and had a tag around his neck that indicates this. It is presumed that his blood sugars are falling.

1. What are some other symptoms of low blood sugar?
2. What is the next step in managing this patient?
3. What are the reasons that his blood sugars would be so low, and how could this be avoided?
4. Does he require evacuation?

Diabetes

The two primary emergencies that can arise in diabetics are very high and very low blood sugar. Diabetic emergencies are common in the outdoor setting as diabetics frequently exert themselves too much, don't stay well hydrated, and are not as careful about their food intake.

[handwritten: monitor sugar / insulin balances]

Symptoms of **low blood sugar** include the following: *[handwritten: hypoglycemia]*

[handwritten: brain starts running out of sugar]

- Rapid onset of confusion, irritability, or combativeness
- Hunger
- Normal or rapid pulse
- Normal or shallow breathing
- Pale, sweaty skin
- Loss of coordination, tremors, slurred speech
- Generalized weakness
- Headache, dizziness, and possible seizures

[handwritten: RAPID onset]
[handwritten: you can rub sugar into gums]
[handwritten: Never inject someone w/ insulin ever]
[handwritten: feed complex + simple sugars]

Symptoms of **high blood sugar** include the following: *[handwritten: hyperglycemia]*

[handwritten: – not as dangerous]
[handwritten: sugar isn't getting into cells]

- Slow onset of confusion and irritability
- Hunger and thirst, frequent urination
- Headache
- Blurred vision
- Nausea and vomiting
- Fruity smelling breath and urine

[handwritten: → Hydrate]
[handwritten: smell like they're drinking]

Diabetics almost always have a blood sugar monitor, which can help determine how high their sugar level is. The diabetic should educate additional personnel on how to use their glucose monitoring equipment in case they are unable to measure it themselves. If a diabetic is found unconscious, it is likely a diabetic with low blood sugar, not high.

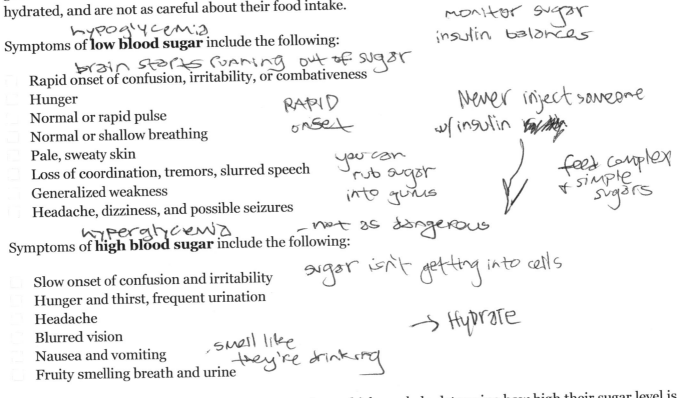

High Altitude and Diabetes

Not much has been written on the topic of diabetes and climbing, although there are more than thirty insulin-dependent diabetics worldwide who have spent time at altitudes above 5000 meters. Diabetics have climbed 8000 meter peaks and have climbed the biggest walls in the world. Stable diabetics can travel safely to high altitudes if they are comfortable with self-monitoring and are willing to pay closer attention than usual to their sugar balance.

Treatment

The treatment for **low blood sugar** includes:

- Sugar – any form of sugar will be sufficient, including candy, sports drinks, starchy foods, etc.
- If the patient is unconscious, sugar (in any form) can be rubbed or poured carefully onto the gums.
- This is a true medical emergency that needs treatment in the backcountry setting.
- Evacuation should be considered depending on how quickly the patient recovers, as well as the difficulty and length of the evacuation process.

The treatment for **high blood sugar** includes:

- If the patient is comfortable managing mild elevations in their blood sugar using previous recommendations by their physician, that is OK. Just make sure they are monitoring their sugar closely. If there is no significant change after several hours, the patient may need to be evacuated.
- Very high blood sugar needs to be treated, but there are usually several hours to get definitive care since the brain has an adequate supply of sugar. Be careful about giving extra insulin to these patients because you do not want to overshoot and make them hypoglycemic. Most patients have a sliding scale that they utilize to keep their serum glucose at an appropriate level.
- Make sure the individual consumes lots of fluids. When blood sugar is high, the patient will urinate often, potentially leading to dehydration. Do not hydrate with only water. Alternate with very diluted sports drinks to help replace important electrolytes. The small amount of sugar found in diluted sports drinks will not make a significant impact on high blood sugar levels.

Prevention is the key to treatment of diabetic problems. The following guidelines will help the well-controlled diabetic to avoid emergencies in the backcountry:

- Ask anyone with diabetes to be free of "crashes" for at least one year.
- Make certain that diabetics have an adequate supply of their medicines (at least twice as much insulin as needed).
- Make sure the diabetic is aware of or has participated in the rigors of the outdoor environment.
- Keep all patients with diabetes well hydrated, even more than the average person.
- Keep a source of sugar nearby.
- Remember that insulin has a very narrow temperature range for it to be effective and must be kept cool.

ALLERGIC REACTIONS AND ANAPHYLAXIS

Case 5

You are biking on trail east of small city. You come across a 17-year-old female who is on the ground with a number of people gathered around her. She is having difficulty breathing and states she was stung by a bee while riding. She has a history of severe allergies to bee stings.

1. What is the most likely diagnosis of this patient?
2. What medicines should this patient receive?
3. Does she require evacuation?

Types of Reaction

There are two main types of allergic reactions: local and general.

Local

Local allergic reactions are characterized by these symptoms:
- Swollen and reddened area(s) of the skin
- Itchy (and sometimes painful) area(s) of the skin

General

Generalized allergic reactions many have the same symptoms as the local reaction in addition to any combination of the following:
- Urticarial rash (commonly known as hives)
- Swelling to the face, arms or legs
- Nausea and vomiting
- Diarrhea

Any of these may begin hours after the exposure to the offending agent occurs. Generalized reactions may progress to a condition called anaphylaxis, which is a serious life-threatening emergency. Symptoms of anaphylaxis include any of the above in addition to the following:

- Shortness of breath and wheezing
- Lightheadedness (from dropping blood pressure)
- Swelling of the tongue and lips, airway constriction
- Confusion
- Painful tightness in the chest
- Loss of consciousness

Treatment

Local reactions:

- Cold packs may alleviate some of the irritation.
- Scratching should be minimized as it may open the area up to infection.
- Topical corticosteroids such as hydrocortisone cream can be helpful in relieving the symptoms.
- Over-the-counter antihistamines such as Diphenhydramine (Benadryl®) may be useful but can also cause drowsiness.

Generalized reactions:

- If it is known what the patient is allergic to, they should be removed from the source immediately (i.e. if they are allergic to bees, the victim should be protected from further stinging, etc.).
- If over-the-counter Diphenhydramine is available, it should be administered immediately. This may slow/prevent the anaphylactic reaction.
- If any respiratory symptoms are present, an EpiPen® or equivalent epinephrine auto injector should be administered. The wilderness medicine guide should be prepared to administer this medication if it is available.
- Any patient with symptoms of anaphylaxis should be evacuated, even if they improve with initial treatment.

Prevention

- If a member of the group entering the backcountry has a known severe allergy to something they may be exposed to while in the wilderness, they must carry an epinephrine auto injector and Diphenhydramine.
- Epinepherine auto injectors can be obtained by the individual with allergies from their physician prior to entering the backcountry.

ABDOMINAL EMERGENCIES

Case 6

You are on a multi-day hike in the wilderness with several people. One member of your party, a 22-year-old female, starts complaining of some lower abdominal pain. She denies fever and constipation, but does state some nausea. When asked about her last menstrual period, she states she "always has irregular periods." She wants to continue hiking but says the pain seems to be getting worse.

1. What concerning features does this patient present with?
2. What easy-to-carry test might be helpful in this case?
3. Should this patient be evacuated or would observation be prudent?

Abdominal Pain

The exact cause of abdominal pain can be very difficult to determine, especially in the backcountry setting. There are many life-threatening causes as well as many benign causes of abdominal pain. In general, certain features of a patient complaining of abdominal pain should alert the wilderness medicine provider to a possibly serious cause:

- Pain with fever and chills
- Pain with vomiting
- Worse pain with movement (as opposed to no change in pain with position changes or walking)
- Pain in a pregnant female
- Pain in a female with unknown pregnancy status
- Blood in the stool, urine, or vomit
- Prolonged pain after trauma to the abdomen
- History of multiple previous abdominal surgeries
- History of previous ectopic pregnancy (pregnancy outside the uterus)

Common Causes in the Wilderness:

- Food poisoning (gastroenteritis)
- Dehydration leading to constipation
- Ectopic pregnancy
- Kidney stones
- Gallstones

Treatment

The primary goal of the wilderness medicine provider is to make the patient comfortable and try to determine if the patient should be evacuated.

Prevention

In general, it is difficult to "prevent" most causes of abdominal pain in the wilderness. Some things that can be done to help prevent an unnecessary evacuation include the following:

- Carry a pregnancy test on a multi-day trip when females of childbearing age will be participating. A pregnancy outside the uterus (or ectopic pregnancy) is a serious life-threatening condition that cannot be diagnosed outside the medical setting. Unfortunately, most sexually active women are not able to accurately determine if they are pregnant or not, even if they believe themselves to be at little or no risk. A female with abdominal pain and a positive pregnancy test needs immediate evacuation.
- Use appropriate water filtration devices. Contaminated water can lead to severe abdominal pain, vomiting and diarrhea.
- Maintain adequate hydration, and carry appropriate foods or medications to prevent constipation. Severe constipation can cause abdominal pain and may mimic more severe causes of pain.

MEDICAL EVACUATION GUIDELINES

Abdominal Problems

When patients receive serious abdominal injuries, they need to be evacuated immediately.

General Evacuation Guidelines:

Evacuate if abdominal pain is accompanied by of the following conditions:
- The pain persists for longer than 24 hours.
- Blood appears in the vomit, feces or urine.
- The pain is associated with a fever.
- The pain is associated with pregnancy.
- The patient is unable to drink or eat.

Allergy Problems

Patients with symptoms of anaphylaxis or severe generalized allergic reaction should be evacuated for further medical evaluation.

Chest Pain

Patients with concerning historical features or symptoms as listed above should be evacuated for further medical evaluation. If there is any doubt, the patient should be evacuated.

Diabetic Emergencies

- Patients with high blood sugar should be evacuated if treatment is not working.
- Patients with low blood sugar should be evaluated for evacuation based on effectiveness of treatment and patient's wishes.

Neurologic Emergencies

- Evacuate any patient suffering a stroke, a TIA (minor stroke), or a new seizure.
- A significant change in mental status should lead to patient evacuation.

Shortness of Breath

- Patients complaining of shortness of breath with concerning historical features or symptoms, or those who do not improve with a brief period of rest should be evacuated immediately.
- Patients with known asthma need to be evacuated if their symptoms are not easily controlled with their own medications.

PREVENTION OF INFECTIOUS DISEASES

Proper hygiene and sanitation practices are essential in preventing infectious diseases of the GI tract. The wilderness traveler must be vigilant to ensure that food and water do not become contaminated. The following guidelines are recommended:

Diet

- Wash hands thoroughly with soap or hand disinfectant before preparing and eating meals.
- Cooking and eating utensils should be cleaned with boiling water or bleach solution prior to each use.
- Avoid raw or undercooked meat, fish and seafood.
- When traveling internationally, avoid street vendors, raw vegetables, and fresh salads.
- Avoid unpasteurized milk, cheese, and other dairy products.
- Peeled fruits and vegetables are generally safe.
- Do not rinse food in water that isn't disinfected.

Water

- Use appropriate methods of water treatment.
- When traveling internationally, avoid tap water and ice cubes made from untreated water.
- Purchase name brand bottled water, and always check the seal prior to drinking.

EVACUATION GUIDELINES

- Any patient with moderate to severe abdominal pain that does not improve over 12-24 hours should be evacuated.
- Patients unable to take sufficient oral rehydration fluids for more than 24 hours should be evacuated.
- Anyone experiencing mental status changes, signs of significant dehydration, hematemesis, or copious bloody stools should be evacuated immediately.
- Patients with signs and symptoms of dysentery who do not respond to appropriate antibiotic therapy in 24-48 hours should be evacuated.

QUESTIONS

1. **A member of your hiking party approaches you and states he is having some chest pain. Which of the following would not be a major concerning feature of his pain?**
   a) History of diabetes
   b) Pain is described as sharp and radiates to his right arm
   c) Associated shortness of breath
   d) The patient is 52-years-old
   e) The pain gets worse with exertion

2. **Which of the following patients with a history of asthma should be evacuated?**
   a) 33-year-old female whose symptoms resolve with a single use of her inhaler and do not recur
   b) 24-year-old female who forgot her inhaler on a day hike but is not having symptoms
   c) 37-year-old male on a multi-day rafting trip with wheezing, fever, and productive cough whose asthma symptoms respond to his inhaler
   d) 18-year-old male who uses his inhaler twice in one day during a multi-day hike

3. **While taking a break on a long single-track mountain bike course, your friend begins to have a seizure. He has never had seizures before as far as you know. Which of the following should NOT be performed during his seizure:**
   a) Avoid placing objects in the patients mouth
   b) Clear the immediate area around him
   c) Avoid holding him down
   d) Roll him on his side after the seizure has finished
   e) All of the above should be performed

4. **Symptoms of HIGH blood sugar include all of the following except:**
   a) Coma
   b) Fruity smelling breath and urine
   c) Nausea and vomiting
   d) Frequent urination
   e) Headache

5. **Prior to going for a multi-pitch climb in a national park, a member of your party states she has a severe allergy to bee stings. Your advice to her should be:**
   a) No problem, there won't be any bees
   b) Just take some Benadryl® before we go, shouldn't be an issue
   c) You should get an epinephrine auto-injector from your doctor before we go
   d) Just bring some Benadryl® with us in case you get stung
   e) We should cancel the trip

ANSWERS
1. d 2. c 3. e 4. a 5. c

CHAPTER 21
Musculoskeletal Injuries

This chapter describes how to recognize, treat, and prevent injuries to the musculoskeletal system.

- Be able to properly use the medical terms of sprain, dislocation, open fracture and closed fracture
- Be able to properly manage dislocations, strains, and sprains
- Recognize signs and symptoms of simple and open fractures
- Understand and demonstrate proper splinting techniques
- Describe when and how you would realign and splint fractures in the wilderness setting
- Identify and treat life-threatening musculoskeletal injuries

TYPES OF MUSCULOSKELETAL INJURIES

General Guidelines

- Consider the mechanism of injury as this will help with the diagnosis.
- Examine the area for point tenderness, swelling and discoloration.
- Examine the range of motion of the injured joint, if the patient can tolerate this, it might be possible to use the injured joint.
- The most important factor is the patient's ability to use the injury

☐ Can the patient complete the wilderness activity?
☐ Is the patient able to walk to definitive care?

RICES for Treatment

RICES is the acronym that is used to treat sprains: Rest, Ice, Compression, Elevation, and Stabilization. This treatment helps to prevent/reduce swelling.

Follow the RICES treatment for the first 72 hours following the injury.

☐ **Rest:** Rest the joint from activity and stress. Immobilize it if necessary.
☐ **Ice:** Apply ice or cold packs for 15-20 minutes, which should be repeated at the rate of about twice an hour.
☐ **Compression:** Follow the ice with a compression wrap. The wrap should compress the joint, but not so tightly that it restricts circulation.
☐ **Elevate:** Elevate the joint above the level of the victim's heart to minimize swelling.
☐ **Stabilization:** Tape or splint the injured joint for transport.

Tendonitis

This is the inflammation of a tendon because of overuse

This is very common in such sports where the participant will use a tendon over and over such as in paddling or hiking

These can be very annoying or completely limiting.

Treatment of Tendonitis

The best treatment is to decrease the use of the joint
This might be impossible given the circumstances
RICES therapy
Anti-inflammatory drugs help considerably

Sprains

A sprain involves the ligaments (tissue that connects bone to bone) of a joint and means that the ligaments have been stretched or even torn.

A sprain usually occurs when a joint is twisted or wrenched beyond the normal range of motion that causes the ligaments to stretch or tear.

While sprains can occur in any joint in the body they happen most often in the knees and the ankles. Symptoms include pain, swelling, and discoloration of the injured joint.

Sprains can be difficult to differentiate from fractures, due to the fact that they share many of the same signs and symptoms.

They are usually graded from 1 – 3

☐ Grade 1: ligament is not torn, little swelling and generally stable
☐ Grade 2: ligament partially torn, more swollen, discoloration from bleeding
☐ Grade 3: ligament torn, very swollen, tender and significant discoloration

Treatment of Sprains

- RICES therapy
- Patient's frequently cannot use the affected joint
- May need help to walk if this is a knee or ankle – litter evacuation may be needed

Strains

- Strains, unlike a sprain, involve tendons that are the fibrous bands that connect muscles to bones and facilitate the movement of our limbs.
- A strain, simply put is fatigue due to overuse or strenuous movements.
- While strains are usually considered to be minor injuries, they can cause pain and discomfort.

Treatment of Strains

- RICES therapy
- The best way to deal with strains is to try and minimize the use of the limb that is causing pain.
- Anti-inflammatories as well as analgesics can help to combat both the inflammation and pain that accompany strains.

Dislocations

- A dislocation occurs when a sufficient force (a push or a pull) is placed on a joint that causes a bone to come out of its socket.
- Dislocations are most common in the shoulder, elbow, finger, and kneecap.
- While dislocations themselves can create quite an ordeal the real damage is usually caused to blood vessels, nerves, muscle, and ligaments.
- Signs and symptoms of a dislocation include:
  - ☐ Severe pain within and deformity of a joint. Deformity is usually very evident.
  - ☐ Inability to move a joint because of pain.
- Our bodies are symmetrical so comparing a joint to the uninjured side may be helpful in being able to determine if a dislocation has occurred or not.

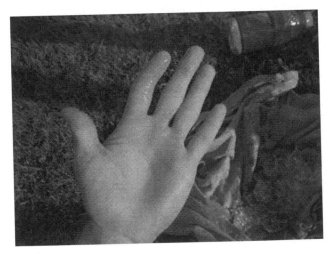

Figure 21.1

Treatment of Dislocations

- After a dislocation occurs the muscles that surround the joint will begin to spasm making it harder to reduce the dislocated limb.
- This makes reduction more difficult with time
- If you know how to reduce a dislocated limb, then the sooner after the injury it is attempted the higher the chance that you will be able to reduce.
- Reducing a limb will also be helpful to the victim as dislocations are very painful and reducing them can provide relief.
- Transporting an injured patient is easier as well
- Probability of damage to nerves and circulator systems is lowered

Reduction

- Use as many resources as possible
- Place yourself comfortably
- Take a firm grip distal to the injury and provide traction-in-line
- Pull steadily, increasing pull slowly, and not jerking
- Gently move extremity toward normal alignment, do not use force.
- Stop if pain increases, most patients will feel relocation take place and feel relief

After Reduction

- Splint the joint with plenty of padding.
- Ice the joint to minimize swelling.
- Check for sensation and circulation distal to the injury.
- Most dislocations should be evacuated for definitive medical care
- Dislocations that resist reduction should be evacuated immediately
- Dislocation of fingers or toes and chronic dislocations don't need to be evacuated if joint is usable

Fractures

- A fracture is any break or crack in a bone.
- There are two general types of fractures:
  - ☐ Closed fracture: In this case the bone is broken but has not punctured the skin exposing the bone.
  - ☐ If a closed fracture is left untreated or handled improperly, it can quickly progress into an open fracture.
  - ☐ If you suspect a bone fracture DO NOT try to move the suspected injury to test for pain.

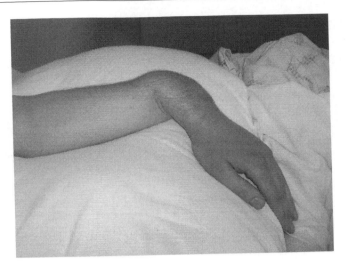

Figure 21.2 – Closed fracture "false joint"

☐ Open (compound) fracture: Just like a closed fracture the bone is broken except in this case the fractured bone has punctured the skin creating an open wound.

☐ Be aware that the bone does not need to be protruding out to be considered an open fracture.

☐ This may happen when the broken bone cuts through the skin, or when an object breaks the skin as it fractures the bone.

☐ Open fractures can be much more cause for alarm due to the fact that the open wound allows bacteria as well as other foreign debris into the body.

☐ Such bacteria and debris can ultimately lead to serious bone or other tissue infection that can impede bone and wound healing.

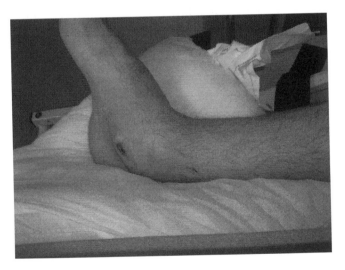

Figure 21.3

■ Since fractures can be difficult to diagnose without x-rays the following signs may help to indicate where there is a fracture.

■ Note that even with these guidelines it will not be possible to identify all bone fractures.

    ☐ Point tenderness - pain and tenderness at a very specific point of the body.

☐ Deformity – as mentioned before our bodies are symmetrical so if there is an abnormal shape position, or motion of a bone/joint then a fracture could be present.

☐ Inability to use the extremity – a bone fracture can most likely render the limb unusable. If a victim cannot move the limb or joint, or cannot bear weight on it, a fracture should be suspected.

☐ Swelling and bruising – at or around the fracture site.

☐ False joint – the ability to move a limb at a point where no joint formally exists.

☐ Bone snap – sometimes the victim will hear or feel a bone snap which can help to diagnose a bone fracture.

☐ Crepitation - the grinding of bones that can sometimes be heard moving a fractured bone.

As mentioned before, a sprain and a fracture are sometimes difficult to differentiate. If you are not sure which injury the victim has splint the extremity and assume it is fractured.

Treatment of Fractures

Since fractures and dislocation injuries are very serious injuries it is important to thoroughly examine them. Here are some general guidelines to help in the process of diagnosing a musculoskeletal injury:

If the mechanism of injury is unknown or such that a neck or back injury is suspected, immobilize the neck immediately upon reaching the victim.

Completely uncover the injured area to look for deformity, swelling, discoloration, breaks in the skin consistent with an open fracture, and other associated injuries.

Gently feel the injured area for tenderness, abnormal movement, and crepitation.

Check for numbness or altered sensation beyond the injury.

Check circulation beyond the injury by pinching the fingernail or toenail bed (if the injury is to an arm or leg) and see how long it takes for the color to return to normal (from white to pink). It should be less than 3 seconds.

Splinting Basics

The main reason for splinting an injury is to immobilize a limb so as to not exacerbate an injury

Splints can also help to reduce pain that accompanies various musculoskeletal injuries.

It is also only a preliminary treatment prior to evacuating a victim to seek further medical care.

General principles regarding splinting include:

☐ A splint should be long enough to immobilize the joints both above and below the fracture, sprain or site of dislocation

☐ The splint should immobilize the fractured limb in its functional position.

☐ The leg should be splinted with a slight bend at the knee.

☐ The ankle and elbow should be splinted with the joints flexed at a 90-degree angle.

☐ The wrist should be splinted straight or slightly bent backwards (extended).

☐ The fingers should be bent in a position similar to that of holding a can of soda and should have loose swath or cloth in between each finger to ensure proper blood as well as lymph flow.

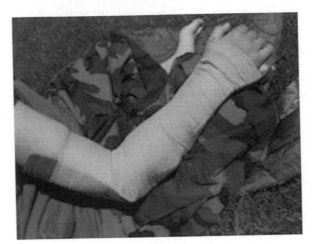

Figure 21.4

General guidelines for splinting include:

Remove ALL (including sentimental) jewelry and accessories, such as watches, bracelets, and rings, before applying a splint. Swelling due to injury will make these objects very hard to remove if left in place.

Use padding within the splint to make it as comfortable as possible for evacuation. Use plenty of padding at bony protrusions, such as elbows, knees, and ankles.

Splints should be made from rigid, sturdy material. Examples are sticks, boards, skis, paddles, heavy cardboard, and rolled up magazines or newspapers. Be creative when creating trying to conjure materials for a splint. Soft metallic splints are a must for any outdoor first aid kit.

Secure the splint in place with pack or lifejacket straps, tape, belts, strips of cloth, webbing, or rope. Tie securely, but not tightly enough to inhibit distal function or blood flow to the limb. Secure the splint in several places, both above and below the fracture, sprain or dislocation. Do not secure a splint directly over the injured area as this can exacerbate the injury.

Avoid moving the injured area unnecessarily.

Mold the splint on the uninjured limb or body part first and then transfer it to the correct site.

After splinting, elevate the injured body part to minimize swelling.

Always recheck distal sensation and circulation beyond the site of injury after placing a splint. If distal sensation and circulation is inhibited due to splinting redo the splint.

Frequently check circulation distal to the injury and splint. If circulation is or begins to be inhibited loosen or reposition the splint to allow proper blood flow.

Realignment of a Closed Fracture

It is not necessary to realign a fractured limb unless distal function and circulation is restricted or in the case that deformity makes it impossible to splint and transport. However, if it can be easily realigned here are some things to consider:

Numbness, tingling, and/or blue discoloration of the skin beyond the injury, all of which indicate poor blood flow (circulation) indicate the need to realigned the fractured limb.

Realignment is easier if it is done soon after the injury, as pain will make it more difficult.

Realignment of a closed fracture can be accomplished by:

Straighten the limb by pulling on it below the fracture in a direction that will straighten it. This should be done while someone else holds the limb above the fracture.

☐ While continuing to hold the limb straight, apply a splint to prevent further motion.
☐ Check distal function and sensation after realignment often and track the limb's progress.

Realignment of an Open Fracture

Reasons for realigning an open fracture are fundamentally the same as for realigning a closed fracture. The procedure for aligning a closed fracture is similar to an open fracture but also includes the following:

☐ The wound and extruding parts of the bone should be thoroughly irrigated and removed of all foreign matter. Although risk of infection is present, it may be necessary to replace the exposed bone end back into the wound during traction for proper realignment.
☐ While continuing to hold the limb straight, apply a splint to prevent further motion.
☐ Cover the wound with a sterile dressing, then bandage.
☐ Check and recheck distal function, sensation and function often after realigning an open fracture.

SPECIAL CONSIDERATIONS

☐ Pelvic and femur fractures are considered worse because of the risk of injuring blood vessels in that area of the fracture.
☐ If these vessels are cut then a person could bleed to death. Special care is to be taken.

Pelvic Fractures

☐ Pelvic fractures call for immediate helicopter evacuation. Arrange for helicopter transport.
☐ Place a sweatshirt or jacket around the pelvis and create a knot that gently secures the fractured pelvis into place.
☐ In the most comfortable position for the victim create a splint by placing padding between the legs and then by strapping the legs together.
☐ Do not elevate the legs.
☐ Refrain from pressing on the pelvis more than as absolutely necessary.

Femur Fractures

☐ Use a traction splint if available. The traction splint will pull the overlapped bone ends into alignment and help to relieve pain.
☐ If a traction splint is not available, then splint the injured leg to the good leg by tying them together and recheck sensation and circulation in the foot often.

PREVENTION

These are some guidelines that will help to prevent musculoskeletal injuries in the backcountry:

☐ Make sure all footwear fits properly and is in good shape. Ankle and knee injuries are among the most common musculoskeletal injuries reported in the wilderness.

- Ensure backpacks fit properly and are loaded with the heaviest items closest to the back with lighter items loaded toward the outside.
- Nylon straps with buckles should be used to secure items to a backpack. Unlike bungee cords, straps hold items better and allow less excess movement that may cause a hiker to fall.
- Always use proper safety gear with secondary safety systems when participating in dangerous outdoor activities, such as climbing, mountain biking and kayaking.
- When planning a trip into the backcountry always devise a plan in advance on how to treat and evacuate all types of musculoskeletal injuries. This plan includes treatment plans, supplies, and how to evacuate a person should a significant injury occur.

EVACUATION GUIDELINES

Reasons for evacuating victims with musculoskeletal injuries from the wilderness include:

- Sprains that are significant enough to prevent further activities in the wilderness.
- All suspected fractures, whether open or closed.
- Any victim who has loss of sensation or impaired circulation beyond the site of the injury.
- Any suspected fracture that is in an area that would be considered life threatening:
  - ☐ Femur fracture
  - ☐ Pelvic fracture
  - ☐ Neck fracture
  - ☐ Spine fracture
- Any individual who is unable to complete all predicted activities in the wilderness due to a sustained injury.

QUESTIONS

1. **Which one of the following signs or symptoms is not necessarily associated with a sprain?**
   a) Pain
   b) Swelling
   c) Crepitation
   d) Discoloration
   e) Unable to put weight on the arm or leg involved

2. **Which one of the following features defines an open fracture?**
   a) Severe uncontrolled pain
   b) Major deformity at the fracture site
   c) Loss of circulation beyond the wound
   d) Inability to use the arm or leg
   e) Laceration over the fracture site

3. **Life threatening fractures include all but which one of the following?**
   a) Femur fracture
   b) Lower leg fracture
   c) Neck fracture
   d) Spine fracture
   e) Pelvis fracture

4. **You are mountain biking when you come upon another rider who has fallen off his bike. He is holding his left shoulder with his right hand and is in a significant amount of pain around the left shoulder. After examining the victim, you are unsure as to whether he has a dislocation or a fracture. You should perform all of the following except:**
   a) Check for circulation to his left arm
   b) Splint his arm with his elbow straight
   c) Splint his arm with his elbow bent at 90 degrees
   d) Recheck his sensation and circulation after splinting
   e) Apply ice to his shoulder

5. **Which one of the following is a correct way to help prevent ankle, knee, and back injuries while hiking in the wilderness?**
   a) *Load your backpack with the heavy items toward the outside*
   b) *Use your friend's hiking boots regardless of how they fit because it is much less expensive*
   c) *Use nylon straps with buckles to tightly secure your tent and sleeping bag to your pack*
   d) *Wear sandals when carrying a heavy backpack*
   a) *Wear a brand new pair of hiking boots on a 3 day expedition over uneven terrain*

ANSWERS
1. c 2. e 3. b 4. b 5. c

CHAPTER 22

Psychological Consequences of Adventure Travel

This chapter describes how to recognize and treat psychological problems that might arise during wilderness travel.

Objectives:

- Recognize occurrence of a potential dangerous psychiatric condition.
- Know how to prepare for and defuse a potentially dangerous situation in which a member of the group may become stressed.
- Be able to recognize and describe multiple psychiatric illnesses potentially encountered in the wilderness.
- Be able to describe ways to prevent exacerbation of a psychiatric illness while in the wilderness.
- Describe, recognize, and treat common wilderness medical conditions that may mimic acute psychiatric disease.
- Know some medications that are reasonable to take on a wilderness trip, and how to treat different acute psychiatric illnesses.

- Be familiar with evacuation guidelines when faced with an acute psychiatric illness in the wilderness.

Case 1

A 40 year old male, whose wife recently died, asks to join your group on a week-long back-packing expedition through the Sierra Nevada Mountains. He thinks the trip will help him clear his mind of his recent loss. He admits to feeling depressed as of late due to the death of his wife. He has a moderate amount of backpacking experience.

You agree to have him join the group on the trip. On the third day of the trip, the weather is much colder than expected. A snowstorm hits in the middle of the day, and the group has to scramble to find shelter and stay warm. Your friend seems to be even more depressed than before the trip. He starts acting bizarre and paranoid. He is convinced the group is trying to leave him for dead. He does not sleep but sits up all night guarding his tent. His behavior progressively worsens such that he is unable to hike.

1. What condition is this person experiencing?
2. How can the group leader help?
3. How could this have been avoided?
4. Why is this situation dangerous?
5. What factors may have contributed to this man's presentation?
6. Should this person be evacuated?

Case 2

You are the medical expert on an expedition on Denali. Everyone in the group has moderate to advanced skill level, and appropriate experience for the trip. One of your team members is a 42 year-old male who has been complaining of chest pain for the past day. He convinces you that the pain feels exactly like his heartburn. The following day as the group heads towards the final summit, the man complains of worsening chest pain. He appears pale and suddenly drops to the ground. He is pulseless and apneic, so CPR is started without success. He dies in front of the rest of the group in spite of your best efforts.

1. How could this have been avoided?
2. What adverse, long-term consequences is the rest of the group at risk for developing?
3. Should the trek to the summit continue?
4. What can you do to help the group best deal with this situation psychologically?

GENERAL

- More people than ever before are taking part in adventure travel and extreme sports.
- Adventure sports enthusiasts spend millions of dollars annually on equipment, yet much less time and money mentally preparing for their trips.
- Most wilderness and adventure trips proceed without incident.
- Emotional reactions to traumatic accidents by victims and rescuers should be expected.
- Most responses to accidents are normal and tend to be consistent.
- Even the most normal responses to accident and tragedy can turn a well-prepared trip into a deadly one.
- Anyone involved in an accident can benefit from attention to this psychological response. Care for emotional needs are as critical as care for physical needs if the individual is to return to a functioning role in society.
- Survival entails being prepared for the worst, both physically and mentally.
- All expedition leaders should be prepared to deal with tragedy and accident both logistically and emotionally.
- Most extreme athletes and adventure travelers will advise participants to mentally prepare by either playing out potentially dangerous mock situations or even by placing themselves in potentially mentally taxing situation. For example, many Ironman athletes will make sure they bike the 112 miles by themselves to get used to the loneliness.
- There is no substitute for adequate preparation.
- Each person on the trip should be familiar with evacuation routes and guidelines.
- Under the proper circumstances, medications should be available and utilized for the safety of everyone.
- Although uncommon, psychiatric disturbances may occur during wilderness travel.
- Some people will experience psychiatric disturbances because of the stress and a perceived loss of control. These people are unable to adapt, and therefore, decompensate.
- Decompensation can manifest in various ways and with various levels of dysfunction including anxiety, panic, depression, and psychosis.
- Environmental conditions themselves, such as hypothermia, high altitude, and hyperthermia can cause an otherwise mentally stable person to decompensate.

THE STRESS RESPONSE

- A crisis is a crucial point or situation that may be unstable, during which people have to respond and adapt to unusual and sometimes critical changes in their environment.
- Most people feel they have control of the things that go on around them and that life events will always go smoothly. If events do change, most people believe they will be able to easily regain control.
- With an unexpected crisis, most people undergo strong emotional changes and become less certain of their ability to influence what is happening around them. Because of stress and loss of control, people may be unable to adapt and may decompensate.

Sources of Stress

- Stress can be categorized as overt or covert.
- Overt sources of stress are related directly to a significant event, such as sights and smells. Stress can be exacerbated when a rescuer or group leader feels inadequate and under-skilled to handle the situation.

Covert sources of stress include fatigue or other logistics that weaken the rescuer. Rescuers and expedition leader who have high expectations of a smooth rescue or trip may end up extremely frustrated and overwhelmed by the death of the victim.

Normal Response to Crisis

During the flight or fight response adrenaline is released to increase sugar consumption and energy. Physiologically, the heart rate, blood pressure, and blood flow to certain muscles increase. There is also increased stimulation of the central nervous system.

Normal emotional responses are: excitement, frustration, impatience, depression, and anger.

Normal stress reactions can be immediate or delayed. Delayed stress reactions appear hours to weeks, sometimes months to years, after an accident and may be directed inward or outward.

Inward reactions include depression, apathy, and feelings of guilt or inadequacy. Nightmares, nausea, loss of appetite, and headache and can be experienced as well.

Outward reactions typically include irritability, explosiveness, and in some cases, anger with others.

Abnormal Stress Response

Changes in productivity, including decreased concentration, loss of attention span, increased number of errors, memory lapses, and difficulty making decisions.

Recurrent and intrusive recollections or dreams of the event.

Markedly diminished interest in one or more significant activities.

Detachment or estrangement from others or emotionally flat or dull affect.

An exaggerated startle response, sleep disturbances, avoidance of activities that arouse recollections of the traumatic event.

Not oriented to time, place, or person.

Observable motor and physical behavior such as mutilation of self or objects or excessive use of drugs or alcohol.

Abnormal verbal behavior ranging from hopelessness to hallucinations or paranoia.

Incongruent emotional expression ranging from bouts of crying to inappropriate laughter.

PSYCHIATRIC ILLNESSES

Generalized Anxiety

- Anxiety disorders are a spectrum of illnesses in which apprehension, fear, and excessive worry dominate an individual.
- Anxiety disorders are diagnosed in 4% to 8% of the general population.
- Anxiety disorders are diagnosed more often in women than men.
- Signs and Symptoms:
  - [ ] Poor concentration
  - [ ] Irritability
  - [ ] Feeling on edge
  - [ ] Muscle tension, which often can be severe enough to cause the patient to experience diffuse muscular pain.
  - [ ] Difficulty sleeping
  - [ ] Gastrointestinal irritability
  - [ ] Increased heart rate
  - [ ] Restlessness
  - [ ] Excessive worry

Panic

- Panic disorder is a type of anxiety disorder.
- It is usually defined as the experience of recurrent attacks of severe anxiety.
- Both anxiety and panic can be worrisome for acute cardiac disease, which may force evacuation.
- Signs and Symptoms:
  - [ ] A sudden extreme surge of anxiety and dread.
  - [ ] Autonomic instability with increased heart rate, shortness of breath, chest tightness, lightheadedness, sweating, and tremors.
  - [ ] The symptoms develop over a few minutes and may be unprovoked or occur with a phobic stimulus like an accident or extreme conditions in the wilderness.
  - [ ] Sleep deprivation can increase the likelihood of anxiety/panic attacks.
  - [ ] Patients with panic attacks have a persistent concern about having additional attacks.
  - [ ] They may exhibit a significant change in behavior during, and later as a result of, the attack.
  - [ ] Patients with panic disorder can also experience agoraphobia, which is characterized by anxiety about being in places or situations from which they see no escape or from situations in which help is unavailable.

Depression

- People embark upon trips with various expectations.
- A fairly frequent and potentially catastrophic misconception is that all that is needed to improve a difficult or painful life circumstance is a change of scenery or vacation.
- If the person is depressed prior to the trip, the outcome can be disastrous and dangerous for everyone involved.
- Signs and Symptoms:
  - [ ] Decreased appetite with weight loss or increased appetite with weight gain
  - [ ] Loss of sleep or too much sleep

☐ Loss of energy with fatigue
☐ Loss of interest with an inability to experience pleasure at something previously enjoyed.
☐ Irritability
☐ Difficulty concentrating
☐ Difficulty making decisions

Mania

Mania is defined as an excessive, persistently elevated, expansive or irritable mood for greater than a week and at least 3 of the following associated symptoms:
☐ Grandiosity or inflated self esteem
☐ Decreased need for sleep without fatigue
☐ Increased talkativeness
☐ Jumping from one topic to the other
☐ Distractibility
☐ Agitation or increase in goal-directed activity
☐ Impulsivity
Mania can also present with psychosis.
Mania is a psychiatric emergency, and can only be stabilized, not fully treated, in the wilderness.
Unsettling circumstances can exacerbate mania.

Post Traumatic Stress Disorder

Post Traumatic Stress Disorder (PTSD) is a chronic psychiatric disorder experienced by people who have been exposed to a traumatic or life-threatening event. Those at higher risk are also those people with current high stress levels and those with a rigid and meticulous temperament.
Diagnosis should be made by a professional.

Psychosis and Brief Psychotic Disorder

Some individuals may become acutely psychotic after exposure to an extremely traumatic life event or experience.
If psychosis lasts for less than 4 weeks, it is termed a *brief psychotic disorder.*
Precipitants of psychosis include the death of a loved one or a life-threatening situation.
Signs and Symptoms:
☐ Auditory, visual, or tactile hallucinations (the latter 2 more rarely)
☐ Inability to logically communicate in a coherent manner
☐ Delusions
☐ Paranoia
☐ Irritability

ENVIRONMENTAL FACTORS WHICH MAY CONTRIBUTE TO MENTAL INSTABILITY

Hypothermia

- Psychiatric presentations and suicide attempts associated with hypothermia are often misdiagnosed initially.
- Preexistent psychiatric disorders blossom again in the cold in some individuals who have become adjusted and stabilized in temperate climates.
- Leaders of expeditions can become moody, apathetic, uncooperative, and become excessively risk-taking.
- Early in hypothermia, simply losing the effective use of the hands can be devastating.
- Appropriate behavior adapted to the cold, such as seeking a heat source, can be lacking.
- An extreme example is paradoxical undressing.
- Signs and Symptoms:
  - ☐ Impaired judgment
  - ☐ Perseveration
  - ☐ Mood changes
  - ☐ Flat affect
  - ☐ Altered mental status
  - ☐ Paradoxical undressing
  - ☐ Neuroses
  - ☐ Psychosis
  - ☐ Suicide
  - ☐ Anorexia
  - ☐ Depression
  - ☐ Apathy
  - ☐ Irritability

High Altitude

- Virtually any circumstance causing hypoxia can cause alterations in mental status.
- Adverse consequences of high altitude will be discussed in more detail in other chapters.
- Mental status changes can range from etiologies such as acute mountain sickness, to carbon monoxide poisoning, to high altitude cerebral edema (HACE).

Heat Stroke

- Potentially deadly if missed.
- By definition, changes in mental status occur in all heart stroke victims.
- The underlying pathology is brain edema and congestion.
- Central nervous system dysfunction is directly related to the duration of hyperthermia, so misdiagnosis can be fatal.
- Signs and Symptoms:
  - ☐ Confusion
  - ☐ Agitation

☐ Delirium
☐ Hallucinations
☐ Ataxia (unstable gait)

IMMEDIATE CARE IN THE FIELD

Medical care of physical injuries and securing the safety of all party members should take first priority.

Just as one would treat shock in the wilderness, the psychological treatment of anxiety and stress reactions should begin immediately.

Some basic guidelines to follow when managing acute mental illness in the wilderness:

☐ Engage the patient in a calm, rational discussion while maintaining a focus on things that are improving during the rescue or crisis

☐ Listen and identify the specific concerns about which the individual is anxious, and show concern as well.

☐ Provide realistic and optimistic feedback by bringing anxious people back to the here-and-now.

☐ Use behavioral relaxation techniques, especially if the patient is hyperventilating.

☐ Use guided imagery such as talk of pleasant events or places to help reduce pain.

☐ Involve the patient to the degree desired and possible to help actively participate in any decision that must be made.

☐ Talk the patient through any technical skills that he or she must participate in by using simple step-by-step advice.

MEDICATIONS

First choice drugs to reduce anxiety are a class called the benzodiazepines. Their names are diazepam (Valium), lorazepam (Ativan), or alprazolam (Xanax). Side effects include drowsiness. Onset of action can be as short as one hour. Benzodiazepines can be given orally or rectally the wilderness. You can obtain a prescription from a doctor to get these.

SSRI medications such as Prozac, Citalopram, Zoloft, etc. can be used for people with depression, but be aware that the onset of action for these medications can be weeks. They should only be started in the wilderness in rare circumstances. The SSRI medications can make the mania worse, which can be catastrophic in the wilderness.

The mainstay of medications to stabilize acute psychosis and mania.

PREVENTION

Be prepared.

Know the group as well as possible.

Predict adverse events and possibly discuss or role-play responses to adverse situations.

- ☐ Use proper nutrition, avoiding drugs and alcohol.
- ☐ Stay calm while helping each individual choose and implement a part of the plan to resolve the crisis.
- ☐ Provide positive feedback.
- ☐ Understand that people will help on their own time.
- ☐ Keep the message to the group simple.
- ☐ When appropriate, laugh and use humor.

EVACUATION GUIDELINES

Any group member who is a danger to himself or herself or anyone else, must be evacuated immediately. Patients who are psychotic or who appear manic should be evacuated immediately as well. Those patients who appear anxious or depressed should be evacuated as soon as time permits to prevent the symptoms from worsening. Those whom you fear are at risk for PTSD after an accident or event should be evacuated as soon as time permits in order to seek immediate professional help.

QUESTIONS

1. A person is on an expedition when a blizzard hits, and he becomes acutely agitated and nervous about the ensuing events. He cannot sleep and states he feels as if his heart is racing. What psychiatric disorder is he currently suffering from?
   a) Psychosis
   b) Generalized anxiety
   c) PTSD
   d) Heat Stroke
   e) Depression

2. What medication is best to treat the above disorder while in the wilderness?
   a) Lorazepam orally
   b) Antibiotics
   c) Vitamins

3. The 40 y/o male in Case One is suffering from what psychiatric disorder?
   a) Generalized Anxiety
   b) Panic attack
   c) Brief psychotic disorder secondary to depression

4. You observe a group member acting strangely, and taking off his clothes in spite of freezing conditions. What disorder do you not want to miss in this individual?
   a) Heat Stroke
   b) Hypothermia
   c) Panic attack
   d) PTSD
   e) Depression

5. A member of an expedition group becomes acutely psychotic. After considering all of the potential underlying medical emergencies, you determine he is having a brief psychotic episode. How do you want to treat him?
   a) Lorazepam and evacuation
   b) Lorazepam and no evacuation

6. **You are a team leader and notice a person developing depression and anxiety during an accident in which another member fell and broke his leg. What is the best initial step in managing this situation?**
    a) Take care of the broken leg and tell the depressed group member that you do not have time for his nonsense
    b) Leave the member with the broken leg to tend to the other member
    c) Tell the depressed member to turn around and head home by himself
    d) Treat the member with the broken leg while calmly engaging the seemingly depressed individual to help out in any way he is able
    e) Walk away from the entire situation, and let the group fend for themselves

ANSWERS
1. b   2. a   3. c   4. b   5. a   6. D

CHAPTER 23

Skin Disorders

This chapter describes dermatologic situations that may be encountered in the wilderness. After reading this chapter you should be able to do the following:

- Recognize poison ivy, poison oak, and poison sumac
- Be able to recognize and treat the rash
- Describe methods of limiting exposure to these plants
- Describe the recommendations for avoiding sunburn
- Understand the proper use of sunscreen lotion
- Understand the treatment for sunburn

Case 1

A 45-year-old woman takes her hiking boots out of storage and joins some friends for a day hike in the early spring. After returning home from a pleasant, uneventful trip, she develops an unrelenting itch on her right lower leg that subsequently develops significant redness. The symptoms remind her of a rash she had last fall after hiking through some dried brush. Strangely, the rash even seems to be in the same location on that same leg. Last fall she had been diagnosed with poison ivy allergic rash, but this time she had hiked on an asphalt trail and had not brushed against any plants.

1. What caused the rash last fall?
2. Assuming she encountered no poison ivy on today's hike, what is causing the rash today?
3. How would you clean her boots to prevent future reactions?
4. How would you manage her current symptoms?

Case 2

A middle-aged potato farmer is attempting to rid his field of the poison ivy that has caused him numerous outbreaks in the past. He builds a large fire and gathers trash, dead wood, and shrubs. He takes special care with the shrubs and handles them with thick vinyl gloves to prevent an outbreak. As he feeds the shrubs into the fire he starts to develop wheezing and progressive respiratory difficulty.

1. What is causing his respiratory distress?
2. How is he contacting the allergen?
3. What is the emergent treatment for his condition?

Case 3

A 17-year-old boy is rock climbing in the desert with some friends. After lunch he is warm and removes his shirt while the group continues rock climbing through the afternoon. That night he has severe pain, warmth, and redness on his back. The pain is worsened by contact with clothing.

1. What is the most likely etiology for his rash?
2. How could he have prevented this rash?
3. What treatments could relieve his symptoms?
4. What are the short-term and long-term outcomes of sunburn?

POISON IVY

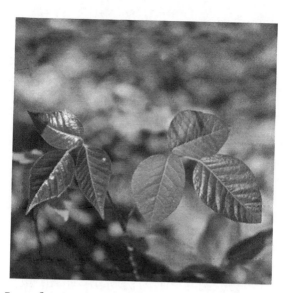

Figure 23.1. Poison Ivy: demonstrating the classical "leaves of three" appearance
Photo courtesy of www.poison-ivy.org

POISON OAK

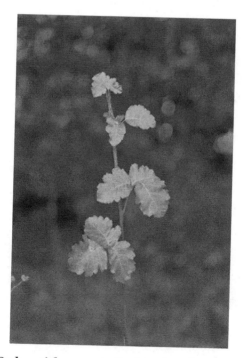

Figure 23.2. Poison Oak: with serrated edges easily confused with typical oak
Photo courtesy of www.poison-ivy.org

POISON SUMAC

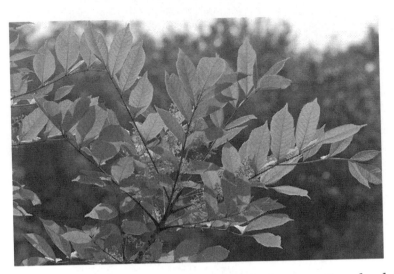

Figure 23.3. Poison Sumac: this deceptively attractive shrub is most commonly found in swampy regions
Photo courtesy of www.poison-ivy.org

POISON IVY RASH

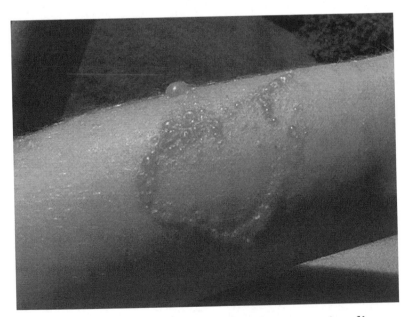

Figure 23.4. Poison Ivy Rash: the classic rash appears in a linear pattern
Photo courtesy of www.poison-ivy.org

Facts

- Poison ivy, poison oak, and poison sumac belong to the *Toxicodendron* genus of plants.
- Exposure to any of these plants causes the itchy "poison ivy" rash.
- These plants grow in every state except Hawaii and Alaska.
- Poison oak, poison sumac, and poison ivy all contain a toxic resin called urushiol, which is responsible for the characteristic reaction.
- Urushiol is a colorless oil contained within the leaves, fruit, root, and stem of the plant.
- Urushiol does not cause the rash unless trauma to the plant releases the resin, but trauma as simple as drying in the fall or raindrops can release the resin.
- Urushiol is remarkably adhesive and can cling to pets, garden tools, and clothing.
- Urushiol is quite heat stable and can attach to smoke particles when the plants are burned, making the potential for airway reactions a frightening possibility.
- The toxin is also very enduring, with reports of the resin causing an allergic rash years after it has left the original plant.
- 85% of the population will develop an allergic reaction if exposed to poison ivy, oak, or sumac.
- Rash may appear after the first exposure, but on subsequent exposures the reaction is more pronounced and has a faster onset.
- People vary in their sensitivity to urushiol. An allergic reaction to the oil can be seen as early as two to six hours in some people or as late as three weeks following exposure.
- Those with extreme poison ivy sensitivity may also cross-react to mangoes.

The Toxicodendrons Plants

- Poison ivy (*Toxicodendron radicans/ rydbergii*) is a climbing vine with **three** serrated-edged, pointed leaves that grows in the East, Midwest, and South. The three-leaf clusters have given rise to the popular adage "Leaves of three: let them be." In the northern and western states, poison ivy is more commonly seen as a low-growing shrub but still with the characteristic three-leaf clusters. Overall, there are many varieties of poison ivy, most occurring east of the Rockies.
- Poison oak (*Toxicodendron toxicarium /diversilobum*) also has three leaves. It grows in the sandy soil of the Southeast as a small shrub. In the western United States, poison oak is a very large plant that grows as a standing shrub or climbing vine.
- Poison sumac (*Toxicodendron vernix*) is a shrub or bush with two rows of 7 – 13 leaflets. It is most common in the peat bogs of the northern U.S. and in swampy southern regions of the country.

Disease Process

- Poison Ivy rash is the term given to the allergic reaction that occurs when the skin contacts the urushiol.
- Urushiol contacts the skin after direct encounter with one of the plants or through contact with a secondary host such as the fur on a pet, a piece of clothing, or even tools.
- Once urushiol contacts the skin, it seeps through the protective outer level known as the epidermis and then causes the characteristic tissue response.
- After the initial exposure, a subsequent exposure may cause a more rapid and more significant response.

Clinical Presentation

The most common clinical presentation of exposure to one of these plants is an itchy red rash on an exposed part of the body (see photo).

The rash often includes fluid-filled small blisters and large blisters in a straight arrangement.

The linear arrangement has led to the misconception that rupturing the fluid-filled blisters while scratching causes spread of the reaction. In fact, the clusters are due to the area primarily contacted by resin from the plant.

The vesicles do not contain urushiol toxin and rupture of the vesicles does not spread the disease.

The rash will only show up in places that come in contact with the urushiol toxin. Therefore, be careful the resin is not on your hands as this can increase the likelihood of spreading.

In a first-time exposure, the appearance of the rash and blisters commonly occurs within 24 to 48 hours but may be delayed up to 21 days.

In a person who has been previously exposed, the rash appears between 4 to 96 hours after exposure.

A small minority of the population is considered "very sensitive" to urushiol. These persons develop the typical itchiness, redness, rash and blisters within six hours of exposure. Other signs such as fever may also appear. These victims need immediate treatment.

Treatment

Early Treatment

Wash the area with soap and water.
- A person can prevent a reaction by washing off the resin within one to four hours.
- Rinsing with copious amounts of cold water will help remove the resin without opening pores or increasing absorption. Avoid rinsing with hot water as it may open your pores, increasing resin absorption.
- Mild hand soaps and non-abrasive rubbing are also recommended.
- Dermatologists suggest repeated, non-abrasive rubbing of the affected area with rinsing in between. Avoid scrubbing.

Rubbing alcohol on a cotton applicator is effective at removing the urushiol resin both from skin and from tools and clothing. Take care to avoid reusing the cotton to prevent spread of the resin.

When cleansing, take special care to remove resin from the fingernails to prevent spreading the sap when scratching.

Mild Disease

Mild rash involves minimal exposure to urushiol and causes small blisters on the skin.

If available, the use of high-potency topical steroid creams before the formation of blisters will offer relief and help to blunt the allergic response.

Avoid the use of high-potency steroids on the face, genitals, and other areas of thin skin.

After vesicles have formed, topical steroids may not change the course of the allergic response but can relieve itching.

Symptomatic relief of the itching can be gained either by using benadary (25-50 mg) or an equivalent dose of another over-the-counter antihistamine.

Several other products are marketed for topical relief of poison rash.
- The skin irritation can be soothed by applying calamine lotion or soaking in Aveeno oatmeal baths.
- Aluminum acetate (Burrow's solution) or Domeboro astringent solution may be applied to help dry out weeping blister for relief of itching.

☐ These topical products offer relief but do not alter the course of the rash.

Topical antibiotics and topical antihistamines should be avoided because these substances have a history of causing allergic rash themselves and may complicate the irritation without offering any advantage. You can identify these topical treatments easily because they typically have the ending "–caine" in their name.

Moderate Disease

Moderate poison ivy rash affects larger surface areas and causes significant distress.

Treatment should include topical steroids if given the opportunity to treat before blister formation.

After blister formation, relief may be obtained by oral steroids for up to 14 days.

A shorter course of steroids may cause a rebound rash that is actually worse than the original illness. In general, the risk of adverse side effects from 14 days of steroids is minor.

Other symptomatic treatment as used to treat mild disease is also appropriate.

Severe Disease

Any reaction that involves the airway, respiratory system, eye, or causes significant genital swelling should be considered severe disease and requires medical evaluation. The most common type of exposure that causes airway or respiratory involvement involves inhalation of smoke from the burning of *Toxicodendron* plants.

If symptoms persist after this time, then IV steroids must be followed by oral therapy as described above.

Disease Course

Most cases of poison ivy rash are self-limiting and resolve in one to three weeks without any treatment.

The vesicles will eventually rupture, crust over, and heal.

Prevention

Avoidance of the *Toxicodendron* plants is the surest prevention of poison ivy rash.

Full-length clothing helps prevent direct contact with the plants, but the urushiol resin can soak through protective clothing if the clothing is wet or the resin is present in a large enough quantity.

Barrier creams such as Bentoquam and other ointments have been marketed to prevent poison ivy rash.

☐ These preparations have varying effectiveness and must be reapplied every few hours to maintain protection.

☐ Bentoquatam (Ivy Block) is safe and is probably the most well studied of these products. It prevents rash in 68% of exposures, but like the other creams, it must be applied to the skin every four hours to maintain protection.

☐ Zanfel is advertised to diminish the reaction if applied early enough after exposure.

■ If in doubt about exposure, wash the exposed areas very well with soap and water.

Do <u>not</u> burn poison ivy, oak or sumac. Breathing the smoke is dangerous

Evacuation Guidelines

The majority of cases of poison ivy rash do not require any evacuation.

Evacuate the exquisitely sensitive victim who develops a severe allergic response.

Evacuate anyone with exposure that involves the eyes or airway or anyone who has respiratory difficulty. These scenarios are most commonly seen with smoke inhalation.

SUNBURN

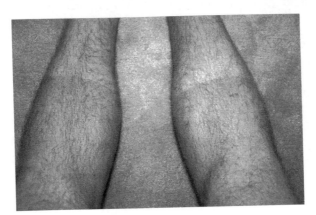

Figure 23.5 Sunburn

Facts

- Sunburn is inflammation / irritation of the skin that is caused by overexposure to the sun.
- Sunburn also predisposes people to skin cancer.
- Ultraviolet (UV) rays from the sun cause sunburn.
- Roughly 32% of adults and 80% of young people reported at least one case of sunburn in the previous year.
- Skin cancer is a serious health problem in the United States, affecting almost a millions each year. Many thousands of people will die each year of malignant melanoma.
- Current studies have shown that 1/65 people will develop malignant melanoma in the world and more shockingly, 1/5 people will develop carcinoma of the skin.
- "Tanning" is UV exposure just like any other sunlight exposure and confers the same risk of skin cancer. This includes tanning-bed UV exposure.
- Fair-skinned people are most susceptible to sunburn because their skin produces only small amounts the protective pigment melanin.
- Although darker-skinned people have a lower risk, they too can develop skin cancer.

Disease Process

- Two types of UV rays are clinically important in sun exposure: UVA and UVB.
- UVA rays penetrate the skin deeply. They contribute in a minor way to sunburn but are thought to play a major role in development of skin cancer.
- UVB rays act upon the skin superficially and play the major role in sunburn formation and wrinkling.
- There are no "safe" UV rays.
- UV rays strike the skin and cause multiple effects.
  - ☐ Skin redness appears as the local blood vessels dilate and inflammatory substances (including histamine) are released.
  - ☐ The tissue changes become apparent as redness develops over a period of two to six hours after exposure.
  - ☐ The UV rays also strike cellular DNA, causing damage that may ultimately result in failure of the cell to self-regulate, which leads to cancer.

Clinical Presentation

- A sunburn is generally clinically obvious with redness in the sun-exposed areas.
- Symptoms can vary from mild redness and warmth of the skin to severe pain and blistering.
- The traditional classification of sunburn includes first-degree and second-degree sunburns.
- First-degree sunburns are those with redness and pain that may peel but heal within a few days.
- Second-degree sunburns also have redness and pain, but they also have blisters and cause systemic symptoms such as fever, chills, and headache. Dermatologists state that a second-degree sunburn nearly doubles an individual's chance of developing skin cancer in the future.

Treatment

First-Degree Sunburn

- The mainstays of therapy are pain control and skin care.
- Pain control can be achieved with acetaminophen or nonsteroidal antiinflammatory medications such as ibuprofen. Benadryl may also offer relief from itching and help the patient sleep.
- Skin treatment can include any of the following measures that offer relief:
  - ☐ Cool soaks with water or moisturizers such as aloe vera
  - ☐ Aloe vera has some anti-inflammatory effects that help soothe the pain and improve healing
  - ☐ Topical pain relief with Aveeno lotion, Prax lotion, or Sarna lotion
  - ☐ Low-potency topical steroids

Second-Degree Sunburn

- In addition to the therapies for first-degree sunburns, these victims may require stronger pain medications.
- Use of oral steroids in severe sunburn has anecdotal support but is not recommended.
- Moderately burned skin should heal within a week, but even one bad burn in childhood carries an increased risk of skin cancer.

Prevention

- Avoid the sun between 10 a.m. and 4 p.m. The sun is more direct during these times.
- Wear proper protection from the sun on cloudy days because UV rays still penetrate the clouds and can cause UV damage. Tightly woven clothing provides the best protection because it blocks a high percentage of UV rays.
- Use waterproof sunscreen on legs and feet when swimming because UV radiation can penetrate through water.
- Wear an opaque shirt in the water because reflected rays are intensified.
- Wear breathable full-length clothing, use wide-brimmed hats, and seek shade.
- When the sun cannot be avoided, sunscreen should be worn.
- Everyone six months of age and older should use sunscreen. Infants younger than six months of age should be kept out of the sun because their skin is thin and very susceptible to burning.
- It is important to understand the proper use and utility of sunscreen.
  - ☐ Traditional sunscreens contain the chemical PABA, which only protects against UVB rays.

- ☐ Newer "broad spectrum" sunscreens contain additives that protect against the UVA rays in addition to the typical UVB protection.
- ☐ Sunscreens are rated according to their Sun Protection Factor (SPF).
  - SPF compares the amount of time to sunburning compared to no protection.
  - Wearing a sunscreen with an SPF of 2 means that a person could stay in the sun 2 times longer before burning than if he or she had no protection. For example, a person who normally sunburns after 15 minutes without protection would take twice that long (30 minutes) to develop sunburn if he or she were wearing SPF 2 sunscreen. That same person, if wearing SPF 10 sunscreen, would take 150 minutes to burn.
  - The downside to relying only on the sunscreen SPF for sun protection is that it only accounts for exposure to UVB rays that cause sunburns. There is no current system available to determine an appropriate amount of sunscreen protection against UVA radiation, this is important because UVA is the radiation most responsible for skin cancer.
  - Traditional sunscreens do not prevent skin cancer
  - Although there is protection against UVA rays with the "broad spectrum" sunscreens, nobody knows what is considered adequate protection.
  - At present, it is important to recognize the limitations of sunscreens and to use additional methods of preventing sun exposure in addition to the broad spectrum (UVA and UVB) sunscreens.
- ☐ Medical professionals recommend waterproof sunscreen with an SPF of at least 15.
- ☐ Sunscreen should be applied to dry skin 30 minutes before sun exposure.
- ☐ Sunscreen must be reapplied after two hours or sooner if sweating or swimming. Even waterproof sunscreen loses effectiveness after about 80 minutes.

Evacuation Guidelines

- ■ Most sunburn victims do not require evacuation.
- ■ Evacuate if the pain or systemic symptoms, such as fever, chills, and headache, cannot be controlled with the medications that are available.

QUESTIONS

1. **Poison Ivy rash can be caused by exposure to:**
   a) The green leaves during summer
   b) The dried leaves during the fall
   c) The stem
   d) The root
   e) All of the above

2. **Appropriate treatment of poison ivy rash includes:**
   a) Topical steroids creams
   b) Topical antibiotic creams
   c) Soaks to relieve itchiness
   d) Topical antihistamines
   e) A and C

3. **Indications for evacuating a person with poison ivy rash include:**
   a) Involvement of the hands, feet, or legs
   b) Involvement of the eye
   c) Previous exposure to poison ivy
   d) Airway involvement
   e) B and D

4. **Which of the following is/are true of urushiol?**
   a) It has seasonal effect, causing symptoms in the fall but not in the spring
   b) Poison ivy is safe to burn as long as it is dried
   c) It is the active resin in poison ivy and poison sumac but <u>not</u> in poison oak.
   d) It readily clings to tools, pets, and clothing
   e) A and C

5. **Which one of the following is true regarding UV light exposure?**
   a) UVB rays cause sunburn, but UVA rays are harmless
   b) UV rays from tanning beds are not harmful
   c) UV exposure causes cell damage that can lead to cancer
   d) UV rays are not a concern on cloudy days
   e) UV rays cannot penetrate water

6. **If a fair-skinned woman normally sunburns after 10 minutes in the sun, how long will she take to develop the same level of sunburn when wearing sunscreen (SPF 30)?**
    a) 30 minutes
    b) 100 minutes
    c) 150 minutes
    d) 300 minutes
    e) 450 minutes

ANSWERS
1. e 2. e 3. e 4. d 5. c 6. d

CHAPTER 24

Water Disinfection and Hydration

This chapter will train you to treat water collected from a wilderness source so that it has an acceptably minimal risk of causing illness.

Objectives:

- Describe various waterborne pathogens that may cause illness from contaminated water.
- Describe three pre-disinfection techniques to initiate the water purification process.
- Describe limitations and techniques for water disinfection, to include use of heat, filtration, and halogenation.
- Understand the concept of basic hygiene as it relates to ways to minimize gastrointestinal illness.

Case

A group of backpackers traverse a difficult ridge in the High Uinta Wilderness. On reaching the other side they are exhausted and thirsty. Having consumed all available water, they search for the nearest stream.

The icy cold waters are reasonably clear, so they fill their canteens and hydration bladders. As one of the most lightweight options, iodine and chlorine tablets were brought for water disinfection. Although very thirsty, the backpackers are careful to follow the directions on the packaging before drinking the water. The remainder of the trip is uneventful.

About seven days later, two of the hikers develop gastrointestinal distress. They both complain of abdominal cramping and watery diarrhea. One of them develops a low-grade fever of 100.1°F, yet her symptoms resolve over the next few days. The other hiker is more symptomatic with nausea, vomiting, and weight loss. After several days, he is admitted to the hospital because of dehydration and requires IV fluid resuscitation.

During his evaluation, fecal specimens reveal microscopic oocysts, but no white blood cells. There are no other specific signs or symptoms. An infectious disease physician orders some specialized tests, which confirm an infection with *Cryptosporidium*.

There is no effective treatment available for this illness; however, the hiker improves with supportive treatment and is discharged from the hospital.

BACKGROUND

The human body depends on a constant influx of water for survival. Gastrointestinal illness from poorly treated water is a major cause of diarrhea and hypovolemia in the wilderness setting. In a survey of wilderness hikers seven days into their trip, diarrheal illness was the second most common medical complaint (56%), closely following blisters (64%).

The goal of water decontamination and disinfection is to eliminate or reduce the number of infectious microorganisms to an acceptably low number.

Unfortunately, merely straining water through a handkerchief and then judging water by its taste, appearance, and location are unreliable methods for determining its safety for consumption. By understanding and practicing the guidelines in this chapter, one should be able to minimize the risk of acquiring waterborne illness in the wilderness.

MICROBIOLOGIC ETIOLOGY

Waterborne pathogens fall into four major categories:
- bacteria
- viruses
- protozoa
- helminths

The likelihood of encountering any of these microorganisms depends on the location and exposure of the water source to contamination.

☐ Watershed areas with animal grazing and human contact have different risks than water that seemingly comes from an underground source. Some organisms may reside in particular soils and contaminate surface water.

☐ As a general guideline, pristine watershed areas tend to be free of viral agents. With increasing human and animal contact, viral contamination becomes more of a concern.

☐ In the field, it can be very difficult to determine who or what has been in the area before you. In order to be safe, one should adhere to the principle that all wilderness water sources are contaminated.

☐ In the past, much attention has been given to the protozoan *Giardia lamblia* as a cause of wilderness gastrointestinal illness. While it is an important organism to consider, some experts believe it is much more likely that bacteria cause the majority of wilderness gastrointestinal illness in North America.

The table below categorizes some of the possible waterborne pathogens:

Waterborne Pathogens

Bacteria	Viral Agents	Protozoa	Helminths
Escherichia coli Shigella Campylobacter species Salmonellae Yersinia enterocolitica Aeromonas species Vibrio cholerae	Hepatitis A Hepatitis E Norwalk agent Poliovirus	Giardia lamblia Entamoeba histolytica Cryptosporidia Cyclospora species Blastocystis hominis Acanthamoebae Balantidium coli Isospora belli Naegleria fowleri	Ascaris lumbricoides Taenia species Trichuris trichiura Fasciola hepatica Strongyloides species Echinococcus Diphyllobothrium species

PRE-DISINFECTION TECHNIQUES

Purification

When water is initially collected, it is important to minimize accumulated particulate matter. Organic and inorganic particles can interfere with the disinfection process, as well as make for an unpleasant drinking experience.

Two of the following steps involve waiting. Depending on the urgency of your situation, you will have to decide if you have enough time and adapt accordingly. It is imperative to understand that these procedures do not disinfect water but enhance the disinfection process and drinking experience.

Screening

This is the process of removing the largest contaminants. This involves using a primary filter as a screen to hold back dirt, plant, and animal matter. Many filtration systems already have a "pre-filter" attached. If one is filling a container by dipping or pouring, he can screen out unwanted debris by pouring the water through a cloth, such as a bandana, handkerchief, or even a t-shirt. One should always include this step in preparations.

Standing

Having the water remain undisturbed for a period of time allows particles that were small enough to pass through the screening material to fall to the bottom of the container. Within as little as one hour, even muddy or turbid water will show significant improvement as the silt settles. After some settling has occurred, the clearer water can be decanted from one container into another, leaving the sediment behind.

Flocculating

This is a method of removing particulate matter that is so small that it would normally stay suspended in water indefinitely. Adding specific chemicals to the water can promote agglomeration of smaller particles until a complex forms that is large enough to precipitate. One such chemical is "alum," which can be purchased from the grocery store. It is also found in baking powder. Add a "pinch" for every gallon of water and then stir it gently for about five minutes. After stirring, allow the water to stand and settle before decanting off the cleaner water.

In wilderness settings, the fine, white ashes from burned wood are rich in mineral salts containing some of these flocculating compounds.

DISINFECTION METHODS

Geneearlly speaking you should always try to use two different methods for treating water. There are several choices depending upon your cirumstances that you can chose

Heat

Enteric pathogens, including cysts and eggs, are readily destroyed by heat. The thermal effectiveness for killing pathogens depends on a combination of temperature and exposure time. Because of this, lower temperatures can be effective with longer contact times. Pasteurization applies this science with carefully controlled temperature. Without a thermometer, it is too difficult and risky to gauge temperature short of boiling.

The boiling point of water is 100°C (212°F). At this temperature, disinfection has generally occurred by the time the water boils. This disinfection has occurred due to the fact that water does not necessarily need to be boiling in order to be disinfected. Because it is difficult to determine the exact temperature of the water, boiling is the safest way to ensure that an appropriate temperature has been reached. One important characteristic of boiling points is that they decrease in temperature with increasing elevation. Some physicians believe this does not make an appreciable difference in water disinfection times. However, the CDC recommends boiling water for three minutes if one is located above 6,562 feet (2000 m).

Using heat properly is a very reliable method for water disinfection. Remember to use a pot cover to preserve fuel when heating water. Also, bring the water to a rolling boil to wash back down any pathogens on the inside of the container and assure the surface of the water has reached the boiling point.

Effective Times for Disinfection Using Heat

Pathogen	Thermal Death
Giardia lamblia, Entamoeba histolytica cysts	After two to three minutes at 60° C (140°F)
Cryptosporidium oocysts	After two minutes at 65° C (149° F)
Enteric viruses	Within seconds at 80° to 100° C (176° F to 212° F)
Bacteria	Within seconds at 100° C (212° F)
Hepatitis A virus	After one minute at 92° C (198° F)

Filters

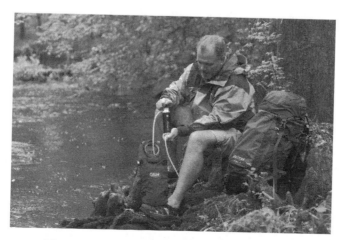

Figure 24.1 Photo courtesy of Katadyn

Filters screen out bacteria, protozoa, and helminths, and their cysts and eggs, but are not very reliable for eliminating viruses.

Viruses tend to adhere to other particles or clump together, which helps remove some of them by filtration. Nevertheless, they are so small (less than 0.1 micron) that they cannot be eradicated by filters alone. Some filters are impregnated with iodine and bactericidal crystals in an attempt to destroy the viruses as they pass through the material. However, these additions are of questionable efficacy.

Because filters work by trapping small particles in their pore matrix, they clog and become less effective over time. Operating a pump as it becomes clogged can force pathogens through it and contaminate the water.

Interpreting advertised specifications for filters can be tricky. The best way to evaluate a given filter is to ascertain its functional removal rate of various organisms. For example, a filter labeled "effective against pathogens" does not truly describe its efficacy. Filters need to eliminate down to the 0.2 micron range (absolute size, not nominal) to be effective for most pathogens, even though larger pore sizes of 0.3 to 0.4 microns may work for many applications.

For practical usage, filters should only be deployed WITH the addition of another disinfection method, unless in areas where human contact is limited and watershed areas are protected. When uncertain, you should use one of the other methods of disinfection as a final step.

Halogenation

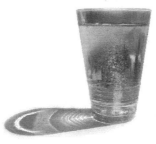

Figure 24.2 Halogen tablet dissolving in water

Iodine and chlorine can be very effective as disinfectants against viruses and bacteria. Halogens are typically faster and more convenient than boiling water. However, their effectiveness against helminths and protozoa varies greatly, and they are more costly. *Cryptosporidium* cysts are extremely resistant to halogen disinfection. The amount of halogen required to destroy these is impractical for drinking.

Regardless of this limitation, the major problem with chemical disinfection is that most people do not perform it properly. Disinfection depends on both halogen concentration and contact time. Factors that affect halogen concentration include water temperature, pH, and the presence of contaminants. Chlorine is more sensitive to these factors, and is thus less suitable for cold, contaminated water. In these conditions, both halogens require increased contact time and/or concentration. Turbid water should be allowed to settle before halogenation because particulate matter can deactivate the available halogen, rendering disinfection incomplete.

Another challenge with halogens is their unpleasant taste. This can be remedied in several ways, but must be done after disinfection. Ascorbic acid (vitamin C) can reduce some of the poor taste. Flavored drink mixes have the benefits of masking some taste and sometimes containing ascorbic acid. Activated charcoal can also be used to reduce the chemical load after disinfection.

There has been some concern that outdoor enthusiasts might ingest too much iodine over a prolonged period. Some studies have demonstrated changes in thyroid function after prolonged use, although the specific amount of time has not been clearly identified. A general guideline is to avoid using high levels of iodine (recommended tablet doses) for more than one to two months. Persons planning extended use may warrant thyroid function studies before leaving and after returning.

For safety, persons with thyroid disease or who are pregnant should not use iodine. People may develop hypersensitivity reactions to iodine.

Other Methods

Ultraviolet radiation (UVR)

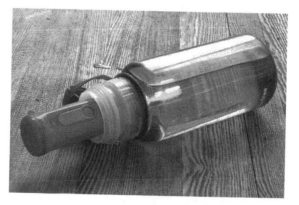

Figure 24.3   Photo by Coronium

UVR has gained popularity as a portable means of water disinfection. Preliminary data show that it can even be effective against the cysts of *Cryptosporidium*. The UV light destroys the DNA of microbes, making them unable to reproduce and cause sickness in humans. Although this method is more expensive, it offers the easiest path to safe water. UVR does have some inherent difficulties, however. It requires a large amount of energy to run a UV lamp and extra batteries are necessary. Additionally, in cold weather, batteries may not be able to provide enough energy to safely power the device. Plus, they are breakable.

Other constraints pertain to water container size and amount of particulate contamination. Particulate matter can act as a shield for the pathogens against the UVR.

All factors considered, this method seems more appropriate for urban international settings than for wilderness travel.

Chlorine Dioxide

Chlorine dioxide has shown promising results. It has been around for quite some time, but has recently been made available for consumer water disinfection. There are both liquid and tablet options on the market.

This substance is chemically different from "chlorine." It is much less reactive with pollutants and has a wider range of effective pH. It imparts much less of an offensive taste than halogens. Additionally, it is one of the only chemical disinfectants shown to be useful against *Giardia* and *Cryptosporidium*.

Summary of Treatment Method Efficacy

Infectious Agent	Heat	Filtration	Chemical
Bacteria	+	+	++
Viruses	+	-	+
Protozoa and cysts	++	++	+
Helminths and oocytes	++	++	-

PREVENTION

Hygiene

As a final note, washing hands and cleaning eating utensils can prevent gastrointestinal illness.

Several studies have shown that hikers are much less likely to develop diarrheal illnesses when they practice proper hygiene. This means using warm, soapy water for cleaning. Being in the great outdoors does not exempt one from hand washing after urination and, particularly, defecation. Eating and cooking utensils should be cleaned thoroughly after each use. Keep your personal utensils out of community cooking gear, and make sure anyone who is sick avoids the food preparation areas.

The same results can theoretically and possibly more easily be accomplished with an alcohol-based hand sanitizer. Remember that hand sanitizer is only effective when there is no visible contamination on your hands. If visible contamination is present, it should be washed away with soap and water if possible.

QUESTIONS

1. **Which one of the following is considered to be the most likely cause of wilderness gastrointestinal illness in North America?**
   a) *Ascaris lumbricoides*
   b) Bacteria
   c) *Cryptosporidium*
   d) *Giardia lamblia*
   e) Viruses

2. **When using heat for water disinfection, the best method incorporates:**
   a) Adding iodine or chlorine to boiling water
   b) Boiling water for 10 to15 minutes
   c) Flocculation of contaminated water
   d) Heating only until the first bubbles start to appear
   e) Screening (filtration) of contaminants before heat treatment

3. **For an extra margin of safety, the CDC recommends boiling water for three minutes above what elevation?**
   a) 3,500 feet
   b) 5,000 feet
   c) 6,500 feet
   d) 9,000 feet
   e) 10,500 feet

4. **Which of the following is the LEAST likely to be found in pristine watershed areas?**
   a) *Cryptosporidium*
   b) *E. coli*
   c) *Giardia lamblia*
   d) Hepatitis A
   e) *Yersinia*

5. **Which of the following is not usually removed by filters?**
   a) *Ascaris* eggs
   b) Bacteria
   c) *Entamoeba* cysts
   d) *Giardia*
   e) Viruses

6. **When choosing a filter, it is important to:**
   a) Choose one that includes activated carbon
   b) Find specific information on the functional removal rate of organisms
   c) Have a nominal pore size of 0.2 microns
   d) Make sure it is "effective against *Giardia*"
   e) Select an "EPA approved" filter

7. **True/False: Filters impregnated with halogens are effective at killing viruses.**

8. **Which of the following CANNOT hinder halogen disinfection of water?**
   a) Adding ascorbic acid or flavored drink mix
   b) Cold water temperature
   c) Halving the recommended dose
   d) Using chemicals before the expiration date
   e) Visible particulate in clear water

9. **True/False: Use of iodine is safe for someone with a pre-existing thyroid condition if it is well controlled by medication.**

10. **Which of the following is the best method for water disinfection:**
    a) Boiling water for 1 minute
    b) Chemical halogenation that properly follows directions
    c) Water filtration with a 0.2 micron absolute pore size
    d) Ultraviolet irradiation or chlorine dioxide
    e) The best method depends on the particular location and group size

11. **True/False: One can effectively reduce the risk of diarrheal illness in the backcountry by properly cleaning hands after urinating or defecating.**

ANSWERS
1. b 2. e 3. c 4. d 5. e 6. b 7. f 8. a 9. f 10. d 11. t

CHAPTER 25

Wilderness Dentistry

This chapter will train you to evaluate and treat oral and dental conditions that occur in the wilderness.

Objectives:

- To understand basic tooth anatomy
- To be able to describe the cause and treatment of tooth pain
- To be able to recognize and treat fillings that have fallen out
- To be able to describe and treat various types of mouth infections
- To be able to describe and treat a fractured tooth
- To be able to describe and treat a tooth that has been knocked out

Case 1

A 38-year-old male is attempting to summit Mt. Denali when he injures a tooth while biting down on a piece of hard candy. He complains of sensitivity to cold and liquids and pain when he bites on the involved tooth, which is an upper left tooth. On examination, you note a missing filling and part of the tooth. There is no bleeding.

1. What is the most likely complication, other than pain, that this climber will have if the tooth is not repaired?
2. What is the best way to repair the tooth?
3. Does this situation require antibiotics?

Case 2

A 56-year-old woman is backpacking in Sweden when she develops a constant ache in her lower left first molar, with sensitivity to cold and pressure. She denies trauma to the tooth. An examination reveals that the tooth has an intact large filling with pain when it is tapped. There is no evidence of tooth fracture or gum swelling.

1. What is the most likely cause for her symptoms?
2. What is the best way to manage this situation, other than pain management?
3. Does this situation require antibiotics? If you were going to use an antibiotic, which one would you select?

Case 3

A 16-year-old climber is struck in the face by a falling rock, which knocks out his right front permanent upper incisor. Fortunately, the rock knocked the tooth back into his mouth, so the victim has the tooth.

1. What is the first step in the management of this tooth?
2. Is this a tooth that should be replanted?
3. How would you clean this tooth if it fell into the dirt?
4. What is the best way to transport this tooth if you do not put it back in?
5. Would your management be different if this was a primary tooth in a 4-year-old male?

BASIC DENTAL ANATOMY

There are three primary regions of the tooth: enamel, dentin, and pulp.

The supporting tissue consists of the gingiva (gum), periodontal ligaments (PDL), and bone.

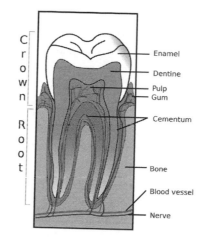

Figure 25.1 Tooth Anatomy

Enamel

Enamel is the outer layer of the tooth and constitutes the crown (part of the tooth one sees when looking in the mouth).

It is the hardest substance in the human body and devoid of nerve endings.

Dentin

The dentin, while still a fairly hard substance, is made up of tiny fluid-filled tubules. The dentin provides nutrients to keep the tooth alive and the ability for a tooth to handle pressure.

If the stress load is too great or a tooth becomes brittle because it has lost vitality, it can break or crack.

If dentin is exposed, a person can experience pain when an applied stimulus makes the fluid in the dentinal tubules move and thus elicit a response from the nerve.

Pulp

The inner layer of the tooth is the pulp chamber, which consists of the neurovascular bundle, often referred to as the "pulp."

When this area is affected, a person can experience pain.

If a tooth is fractured down to the pulp, one may notice bleeding from the tooth.

CLINICAL PRESENTATION AND MANAGEMENT

Pulpitis or toothaches

- Inflammation of pulp tissue (neurovascular bundle) is the primary cause of most toothaches.
- Pain can range from mild to debilitating and can be steady or intermittent.
- The origin of inflammation can arise for the following reasons:
  - Bacterial invasion (consequences of the tooth decay or "cavity" process)
  - Local irritation (e.g., a restoration being placed in close proximity to the pulp chamber)
  - Physical trauma (first causing inflammation of the pulp, and then reducing or eliminating blood supply to the tooth, which causes destruction of pulp tissue)
- Pulpitis in early stages can be reversed. Early on, the tooth will be sensitive to a stimulus such as heat or cold or sweet or sugary food placed on the tooth. Once the stimulus is removed, the tooth returns to its normal state. With irreversible pulpitis, the tooth will frequently remain achy or painful after the stimulus has been removed.
- Pulpitis can be classified into mild, moderate, and severe. The amount of treatment needed varies with the severity of the toothache. Mild pulpitis is often reversible and can be treated simply by avoiding any stimulus. Severe pulpitis requires removal of pulp tissue or extraction of the tooth. This is usually not feasible in the wilderness and therefore warrants evacuation. Until that time, the patient must be managed to reduce pain and to prevent the situation from worsening.

Signs and Symptoms

- Tooth sensitivity or pain to stimulus (cold, hot, sweets)
- Transient sensitivity to debilitating pain
- In early stages, it may be difficult to identity the offending tooth
- Radiating pain may make it seem as if other teeth are involved
- Pain intensity may increase when the victim lies down
- Rarely sensitive to percussion or biting pressure
- Look for tooth decay or a hole in the tooth

Treatment

- Remove any irritant or debris
- Temporarily fill any defect in the tooth
- Avoid stimulus that makes the tooth respond with pain
- Pain management using Ibuprofen for mild to moderate/severe pain and narcotics for more severe pain
- Antibiotics at the first sign of swelling or abscess

Complications

- If dead pulp tissue escapes into surrounding tissue outside of the tooth, the infection can begin to develop into an abscess. Abscesses in the backcountry need to be monitored very closely because of delay to treatment and the possibility of their spreading into deeper and more serious anatomical areas.

Note: If tapping on the tooth with a hard object such as the handle of a spoon causes pain, it means that there is inflamed tissue surrounding the tooth.

LOST FILLINGS

There are several reasons why filling may fall out. With these gone, the tooth may be sensitive or food may get packed between the teeth and irritate and inflame the gums. Temporary filling materials can be used to make repairs until a dentist can be found and a more permanent restoration created.

Lost Filling

Signs and Symptoms

Tooth sensitivity to a stimulus such as cold, hot, or sweets. The tooth is usually fine without any stimulus present.

Missing filling

Sore tongue from rough or sharp tooth edge

Food impaction between teeth, making tooth and gums sore

Treatment

Remove any debris in or around the tooth

Temporarily fill any hole

Temporary filling materiaZs l

☐ There are several commercially available temporary filling materials:
  - *Cavit* comes pre-mixed and will harden once placed in the mouth. Cavit can be thinned, if necessary, by mixing it with petrolatum jelly (Vaseline).
  - *IRM* comes in a powder/liquid form that requires mixing. The advantage of IRM is that it can be mixed to any consistency.

Smooth rough or sharp edges

Complications

Left untreated, bacterial invasion can begin the decay process that eventually leads to irreversible pain and the need for endodontic therapy such as a root canal.

Lost Crown or Bridge

Signs and Symptoms

Tooth sensitivity to stimulus (cold, hot, sweets)

Food impaction around tooth

Treatment

☐ Clean out old cement from inside of crown
☐ Remove any debris around the tooth
☐ Check to make sure that the crown still fits
☐ Place a thin film of soft temporarily filling material in the crown and place the crown back on the tooth
☐ Have the patient bite down to squeeze out excess cement
☐ Note: You may need to thin the temporary filling material if it is too thick
☐ Have patient bite down to ensure that the replaced crown doesn't interfere with his or her bite
☐ Remove excess filling material
☐ Check the bite again

Complications

☐ Left untreated, bacterial can begin the decay process that eventually leads to irreversible tooth pain.
☐ If decay is present under the crown, it may have gone unnoticed. If it is severe enough, the tooth may break off at the gum line and there won't be enough retention to cement the crown back into place. In this case, one could place a small amount of temporary filling material over the remaining part of the tooth to make it smooth, so that the tooth is less sensitive and the tongue won't become irritated.

ORAL INFECTIONS

Mouth infections can be viral, fungal, or bacterial. The first two are less frequent and generally not a major health threat in the wilderness. Bacterial infection can become a serious problem if not treated, in part because they have the potential to spread.

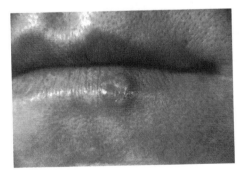

Figure 25.2   Fever blister (cold sore)

Herpes

■ While there are several viruses that have oral manifestations, herpes virus is the one most commonly encountered in the backcountry.
■ Herpes simplex virus generally presents with small blisters in localized clusters, which may come together to form a large lesion.

When the vesicles rupture, they leave a shallow, ragged, and extremely painful ulcer covered by a gray membrane and surrounded by a red and swollen halo. They may form a brown crust on the lips. These are called fiver blisters.

One may reduce the incidence of fever blisters by using sun block.

Symptoms

A tingling feeling
Swollen lymph glands
Sore throat
Low-grade fever

Treatment

Analgesics
Antiviral pills or creams
Soothing mouth rinses, such as warm saline solution
Prevent them by using sunscreen

Fungal Infections

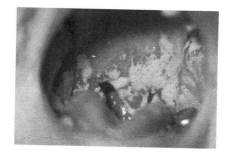

Figure 25.3   Thrush

Fungal infections are most commonly found in individuals who are have low immune systems, or taking antibiotics.

The fungal infection most likely to be encountered is candidiasis, otherwise known as "thrush."

Symptoms

■ White patches in the mouth that can be rubbed off, leaving a raw, red surface

Treatment

Nystatin or a Mycelex Troche

Bacterial Infections

A bacterial infection in the mouth can become a serious health threat. In the backcountry, such an infection should be treated aggressively. Oral infection generally spreads slowly, but rapid spread to deep pockets in the face may occur.

Antibiotics should be started if you can't get to a doctor soon

Tooth Abscess

The swelling of the abscess is confined to the root area of the tooth. Swelling is more common near the jaw and around the infected tooth.

Signs and Symptoms

- Pain
- Swelling (localized)
- Tooth sensitive to tapping
- The affected tooth may be unresponsive to heat because the tooth may be 'dead'
- The patient may have a prior history of a toothache

Treatment

- Pain management
- Antibiotics
- Abscesses need to be opened and drained so getting to a dentist is important.

Antibiotic Use

Mouth infections are usually treated with penicillin. You can also use an antibiotic called clindamycin.

Indications for antibiotic use for oral infections:
- ☐ Antibiotics should be used if delay to definitive care is anticipated.

DENTAL TRAUMA

Injuries to the tooth and supporting tissues are more likely to occur during high-adventure activity mishaps, such as mountain biking, skiing, climbing, or rafting.

Trauma can be isolated to only the tooth but more likely involves soft tissue and supporting tissue as well. Soft tissue consists of the lips, tongue, and cheeks, while supporting tissue is made up of bone, ligaments, and gums.

History and Exam

- Proper evaluation and history are helpful in a trauma situation. In addition to examination of the teeth and surrounding tissue, the victim should be asked about loss of consciousness, nausea, vomiting, and dizziness to identify any possible head injury.
- Clean the region well to unmask injuries hidden by blood or debris. Evaluate lacerations for any foreign material, including parts or pieces of broken teeth.
- Examine teeth for fractures and pulp exposures.
- Evaluate the jaw and facial bones for any fractures.

Injuries to the Tooth

- Tooth injuries consist of fractured or chipped teeth. A fracture can vary from just losing a corner of a tooth to an entire tooth breaking off at the gum line.

Uncomplicated Crown Fracture

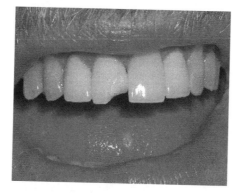

Figure 25.4 Uncomplicated Crown Fracture

Signs and Symptoms

- Visible chip on tooth
- No visible pulp tissue or bleeding
- Sensitive to stimulus (hot, cold, sweets)

Treatment

- Pain management
- Smooth sharp edges by placing temporary filling (IRM, Cavit, soft wax, or tape) over the tooth
- Avoid any stimulus that may aggravate the tooth

Uncomplicated Crown-Root Fracture

- This fracture usually occurs with pre-molar and molar teeth, when part of the cusp has broken away but remains in the mouth because it is still attached to gingiva.

Signs and Symptoms

- Loose piece of tooth
- Pain or irritation on biting

Treatment

- Remove loose fragment
- Cover the tooth with a temporary filling
- Pain management
- Avoid any stimulus that may aggravate the tooth

Complicated Crown Fracture

Signs and Symptoms

- Fracture involving exposure of pulp
- Sensitive to air, cold and other stimuli because of exposed nerve

Treatment

- Stop bleeding by biting on gauze
- Because the nerve has been exposed, the tooth is very sensitive, so the sooner the victim is taken to a dentist, the better
- Cover the tooth with a temporary filling
- Pain management

Complicated Crown-Root Fracture

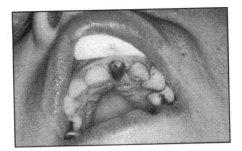

Figure 25.5 Complicated Crown-Root Fracture

Signs and Symptoms

- Fracture that exposes pulp
- Sensitive to air, cold, etc.
- Loose fragment of tooth attached to gum

Treatment

- Remove or stabilize fragment
- Proceed as for a complicated crown fracture

Root Fracture

- This injury may be difficult to differentiate from a tooth that has been knocked out (next section). However, treatment in the field is the same.

Signs and Symptoms

- Slight to severe mobility
- Generally happens to the front teeth

Treatment

- Reposition the tooth and splint
- Pain management

INJURIES TO PERIODONTAL TISSUES

Trauma to the oral cavity may not fracture a tooth. However, damage may occur in the supporting structures around the tooth, in which case the tooth will be displaced from its normal position. The following are possible scenarios that can affect teeth and supporting tissues.

Mild trauma

- The tooth is properly positioned but tender to touch and percussion with possible increased bleeding from gums.
- Treatment consists of a soft diet, rest, and Ibuprofen for pain management, if necessary.
- If the patient keeps biting on the tooth, thus causing pain, have them hold something between their teeth to prevent biting.

Tooth Pushed Into Socket (Intrusive Luxation)

- The tooth has been pushed into the socket. There is no mobility.
- Field treatment is to mange the pain.
- Seeing a dentist should be initiated within two weeks of the incident.

Tooth Partially Knocked Out of Socket (Extrusion Luxation)

- The tooth is knocked partially from its socket and extremely mobile.
- Use gentle steady pressure to reposition the tooth, allowing time to displace any blood that has collected in the socket area. After this is done, the tooth should be non-rigidly splinted.

Tooth Knocked Laterally out of Socket (Lateral Luxation)

- The tooth is displaced laterally because of bone fracture and can get locked into a new position. If this happens, the tooth will not be mobile.
- Push the tooth in using the two-finger technique.
  - ☐ With one finger over the apex, push toward the crown while the other finger places a small amount of pressure outwards to help position the tooth back into its socket. The tooth may snap back into position and be quite stable.
- Splint if mobility is present after reduction.

Tooth Knocked Out of its Socket (Avulsion)

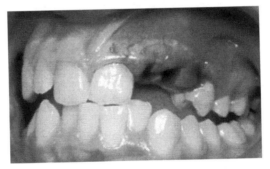

Figure 25.6 Tooth Avulsion

- Quick action is needed to increase survival of the tooth. The longer the tooth is out of the mouth, the less the chance for survival of the tooth.
- Survival also depends on the health of the ligament along the side of the tooth (called the periodontal ligaments or PDL), some of which are on the root of the tooth (others are in the socket).
- Do NOT scrub, scrape, disinfect, or let the root surface dry out; rinse the tooth with salt water to remove debris before replanting it back in the socket. When removing clotted blood from the socket, use gentle irrigation and suction; avoid scraping the socket walls. Replace the tooth gently with steady pressure to displace any accumulated blood.
- If contaminated, rinse the tooth gently before replanting.
- If immediate replantation is not possible, place tooth in the best transportation medium available.
- Transport media (in order of effectiveness):
  - ☐ Save-A-Tooth (Hank's balanced salt solution, which is a physiologically balanced saline)
  - ☐ Milk
  - ☐ Saliva
  - ☐ Saline and water do not work well as transport solutions because they can damage the PDL cells. They should only be used to clean the tooth for immediate replantation and not for transportation.

Management of the root surface:

Keep the tooth moist at all times.
Do not handle the root surface (hold by the crown).
Do not scrape or brush the root surface.
If the root appears clean, replant the tooth.
If the root surface is contaminated, rinse with HBSS or saline (use water if saline is not available).
Persistent debris can be removed with tweezers and then rinsed.

Management of the socket:

Gently rinse without entering the socket; if a clot is present, use light irrigation to remove it.
Do not scrape the socket.
If the bone is collapsed and prevents replantation, carefully insert a blunt instrument into the socket to reposition the bone to its original position.
After replantation, manually compress the bones (only if spread apart).
Splint or stabilize the tooth.

Splinting

Once a tooth has been repositioned back into the socket, it will need to be splinted so that the ligaments can reattach.
There are two types of splinting: rigid and non-rigid.
☐ Rigid splinting is best for the bony segment fractures or jawbone fractures. A dentist usually does this.
☐ Non-rigid is the splinting of choice for tooth stabilization. In a backcountry environment, it may be necessary to improvise with material on hand. Fishing line or even floss could be bonded to splint teeth.

Injuries to Primary Teeth

Primary teeth and baby teeth, are both different terms for the same thing.
When dealing with first aid for primary teeth, the general rule is to remove the tooth if it is in the way.
If a young child has sustained an injury that results in a tooth becoming dislodged or loose, the best treatment is simply to remove it.
It is not necessary to replant avulsed primary teeth. If the displaced primary tooth does not interfere with occlusion, no treatment other than palliative is needed.

QUESTIONS

1. **What is best medium to transport a knocked out tooth?**
   a) Milk
   b) Water
   c) Saliva
   d) Hank's Solution

ANSWERS
1. d (a if you don't have this solution)

CHAPTER 26

Wilderness Medical Kits

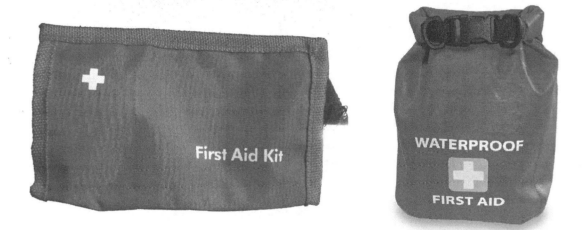

Figure 26.1

Figure 26.2

Bringing appropriate medical equipment and supplies into the backcountry is essential. This chapter discusses general considerations, planning and preparation, and specific items that can be used for multiple purposes.

GENERAL CONSIDERATIONS

With the increasing number of people using the backcountry, the chances are increasing that one with medical training may be involved in providing care in the event of a medical emergency.

The decision of what equipment to bring or to leave behind depends on multiple aspects of a specific trip: type of activity, group size, distance, and time and availability of evacuation. For example, a backpacking trip of seven days over high, mountainous terrain far from civilization requires a medical kit that is lightweight and contains items that can treat emergencies related to high-altitude illness, cold exposure, trauma, geographically specific infectious diseases, and avalanches. This is in contrast to a one-day river trip near a highway where weight is less of an issue and evacuation may be aided by a nearby vehicle. In the latter scenario, a kit with supplies to treat emergencies related to water sports, cold exposure, and trauma would be appropriate.

While having the right equipment is important, it is impossible to carry all foreseeable items into the backcountry. Improvising with what is available becomes necessary for any trip. Items that are versatile or those brought for other purposes such as safety pins, gauze, duct tape, and camping equipment can be used in various ways and can replace specific items.

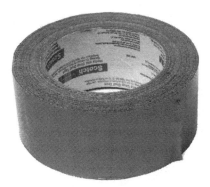

Figure 26.3 Duct Tape

When in a group and especially if you are the medical leader, you need to consider the age, past medical history, and allergies of each member of the group. In addition, everyone should have a kit containing personal medications. The main kit can also be divided among the group.

Keep in mind that people have allergies to medicines and tapes, so bring alternative medicines and supplies.

Several options exist for types of kits. The two most important aspects are protection of the supplies from the elements and organization of the equipment. Cordura is an excellent material for most activities except water-related activities where a waterproof container is necessary. Be careful of the medications that need to be at a certain temperature to maintain their integrity.

Many commercial kits are available and carry essential supplies and equipment but do not contain prescription medications. Making your own kit is another option and can save money. Either way, you will need to make adjustments and bring items that pertain to the specific activity.

SPECIFIC ITEMS

Though it is not practical to list each item that should be placed in every type of medical kit, some general items as well as specific items are listed below. The acronym PAWS, as outlined below, is a way to remember a general guideline of items to place in a kit.

P-Prevention / Procedures

Prevention can make or break a trip and good judgment is the key ingredient. Many crisis situations can be avoided with adequate planning and preparation.

Water filter	Purification tablets	Gloves	Sun screen	Soap
Blister prevention	Insect repellant and barriers	Immunizations for specific destinations	Oral rehydration packets	Extra food and clothing

Procedures require certain tools that may be used in a wide variety of situations. Items in boldface are recommended for a basic kit, while the remainder should be considered for longer trips.

Needles (two to three sizes)	Oro/naso-pharyngeal airway (two sizes)	Safety pins	Tongue blades
Dental wax – filling	Zip-lock bags	Headlamp	Syringes – for medications and wound irrigation
Zerowet for wound irrigation	Scissors	Splinter removal forceps	
12G angiocath + stopcock	SAM splint/ finger splints	Hemostat	Magill Forceps
Scalpel with blade	Needle driver*	Sutures*	Razor
Advanced airway	Bag-valve mask	Epistaxis control- balloon or tampon	Foley catheter

* **Note:** closure of wounds in the wilderness is controversial. For a wound that has a higher risk of infection, delayed primary closure or healing by secondary intention is appropriate. Some wounds may warrant closure for hemostasis or if there is minimal risk of infection. In either case, it is essential to properly irrigate with pressure using sterile saline or filtered water.

A-Analgesics / Antibiotics / Antiseptics

This category comprises medications and other substances for a wide variety of uses in the backcountry. Each member of the group should bring his or her own medications for any preexisting medical problems.

- One consideration for antibiotics is to bring those that cover a wide spectrum of pathogens, thereby reducing the total number packed.

- An antibiotic such as Ciprofloxacin or one such as Azythromycin are two examples that can be obtained from a doctor.

- For analgesia control beyond Acetaminophen and NSAIDs, opioid analgesics may be needed. The oral route should suffice in most instances, but injectable medications may be required. Be aware of the laws pertaining to distributing and transporting these controlled substances as they vary both nationally and internationally.

- Prior to the trip, be familiar with each medication as it is essential to know the dosing, side effects, and contraindications of each one.

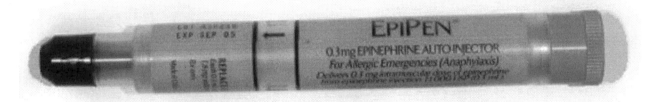

Figure 26.4 EpiPen

Acetaminophen (Tylenol)	Ibuprofen (Motrin)	Diphenhydramine (Benadryl)	Ranitidine (Zantac)
Epinephrine (Epi-Pen)	Glutose paste	Simethicone (Mylanta)	Loperamide (Imodium AD)
Topical steroid	Glycerine suppositories	Azithromycin	Ciprofloxacin
Pseudoephedrine (Sudafed)	Albuterol MDI	Oral rehydration	Aspirin
Amoxicillin with clavulanate (Augmentin)	Ceftriaxone	Metronidazole	Dexamethazone
Analgesic – narcotic oral/intramuscular	Sedative – oral	Acetazolamide	Nifedipine
Anti-malarial/other anti-parasitic	Tinactin antifungal	Prednisone	Aloe Vera
Cycloplegic	Opthalmic antibiotic	Opthalmic anesthetic	Saline eye wash
Antiemetic (oral dissolving or suppository)			

W-Wound Care

This is by far the area that will get the most use, as most injuries are simple wounds. Bring plenty for the small wounds. A wound requiring daily dressings can use up a kit quickly on extended trips.

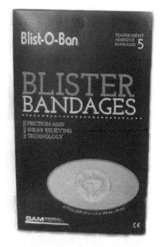

Figure 26.5. Photo courtesy of SAM Medical Products

Gloves	Wound closure strips	Tincture of benzoin	Alcohol swabs
Band-Aids	Moleskin /or 2nd skin	Large trauma dressing	4X4 gauze
Irrigation equipment	Povidone-iodine solution USP 10%	Antiseptic towelettes	Antibiotic ointment
Sterile scrub brush	Knuckle bandage	Sterile dressing	Tape (cloth / duct)
Elastic bandage (ace)	Q-tip	Eyepad	Triangular bandage
Gauze wrap	Tegaderm	Wound adhesive (dermabond)	1% Lidocaine + topical Lidocaine gel

S-Survival

The potential for the group members to be separated and other worst-case scenarios need to be considered. Below is a table of items each group member should have on his or her person.

ID / pencil / notepad	Flashlight	Map / Compass	Matches, lighter
Knife / multi-tool	Nylon cord	Bandana / ace wrap	Energy bar
Gauze / tape	Whistle / mirror	Medications	Space blanket

OTHER MEDICAL KITS

As each trip varies according to duration and type of activity, the kit should be tailored accordingly. Below are a few items that one should bring for a specific trip or situation.

In-vehicle Medical Kit

A medical kit to keep in the car can serve as an extra kit while traveling to a trailhead and as a more comprehensive kit in the event of an evacuation. This kit comprises the previously listed items in addition to the following:

Large burn dressings	Splints, traction equipment	Board for spinal immobilization (folding or short)	Additional gloves
Ropes, rescue equipment	Blankets	Extra food, water	Scissors
Flashlight	Battery cables	Lighter, matches	Long-burning candles
Radio, citizens band	Toilet paper	Tarp	Saw, metal cutting
Foil or window shelter	Chains	Fire extinguisher	Flares (6)
Shovel	Cables / tow chain	Wedgeblocks	Stove, cookware

Specific Activities

Specific activities or certain patient populations may need other equipment in addition to those items listed above:

Climbing and Canyoneering

■ Bring rescue equipment for difficult evacuation, including extra splints, wound care supplies, and water purification.

Mountaineering

■ Bring high-altitude items such as Gamow Bag, extra sunglasses, ophthalmic medications, avalanche safety and rescue equipment, and thermometer. Also, bring cold-exposure materials such as hand and foot warmers, space blanket, and aloe vera (frostbite).

Water sports

■ Bring a bag-valve mask and water purification.

Pediatric

■ Bring medications in chewable or suspension form with the appropriate dosing according to weight, smaller sizes of equipment (mask, airway, and needles), Magill forceps, and tympanic membrane anesthetic.

QUESTIONS

6. **What are the four elements of the acronym PAWS?**
   a) Prevention/Procedures, Analgestics/Antibacterials/Antiseptics, Wound care, Survival
   b) Pulmonary, Aortic, Water, Septic
   c) Pills, Airway, Water, Solids
   d) Pyretics, Anti-inflammatories, Wool, Shovel

7. **What are some examples of items to pack into a medical kit that would help prevent an emergency?**
   a) Road flare
   b) Shampoo
   c) Water filter
   d) Novel

8. **What is the main concern with performing a closure of an open wound while in the wilderness?**
   a) Pain
   b) Infection
   c) Non-ascetic scar
   d) Re-injury

9. **You and several friends are taking a backpacking trip through the Wind River Mountains in Wyoming. Which of the following is NOT an example of something you should bring in a wilderness medical kit in this case?**
   a) Medications for high altitude illness
   b) Medications for cold exposure and trauma
   c) Medications for avalanches
   d) Medications for malaria

10. **Seeing how you cannot carry all items used to treat every foreseeable illness, at times you have to use items that are versatile and can be used to improvise. Which of the following is a list of good examples?**
    a) Duct tape, gaze bandage, safety pins
    b) Portable gurney, surgical scissors, 5L water jug
    c) IV solution, medical splint, 2 pint alcohol bottle

ANSWERS
1. a 2. c 3. b 4. d 5. a

CHAPTER 27

Wilderness Wound Management

This chapter describes assessing and treating injuries to the skin encountered in the wilderness.

Objectives:

- Understand the importance of identifying and thoroughly visualizing wounds in the wilderness
- Describe methods to stop bleeding in a step-wise fashion
- Discuss methods to prevent infection of wounds in the wilderness
- Describe recognition of infected wounds
- Identify wounds that require evacuation from the wilderness

Case

You are backpacking with a group of friends in the wilderness on a multi-day trek. You come across an individual who has a blood-soaked shirt wrapped around his forearm. He states he was free climbing about six hours earlier and fell. You examine his forearm and note an actively bleeding, four-centimeter laceration.

1. How should you examine this wound?
2. What steps should you take to stop the bleeding?
3. What is the most important step to prevent infection?
4. Does he require evacuation?
5. What factors determine the need to evacuate victims with wounds from the backcountry?

ASSESSING THE WOUND

Injuries to the skin are one the most common problems encountered in the wilderness. Due to numerous environmental, wilderness, and supply issues, it can be difficult to properly evaluate and treat a simple wound. Furthermore, once a wound has been treated, it can be difficult to keep an injury, even a simple abrasion, clean or covered properly.

There are general guidelines that can be used to manage any wound:
- History
- Examination
- Control active bleeding
- Cleaning
- Debridement
- Definitive wound care

Before examining a wound, a history of the injury should be obtained.
- When did the injury occur?
- What caused the wound? Was the penetrating object clean or dirty?
- Has the wound been cleaned in any way?
- Is there any chance that a foreign object (e.g., gravel, a piece of tree branch, etc.) could still be inside the wound? Does it feel like a foreign object is in the wound?
- For wounds to the arms and legs: is there any numbness, loss of distal pulse, inability to move fingers/toes, or color changes beyond where the injury appears?

All wounds should be thoroughly examined with a focus on the following areas:
- Type of wound (abrasion, laceration, etc.)
- Location
- Dimensions (width, length, and depth)

Presence or absence of foreign object (dirt, rocks, teeth, etc.)

Other important principles to consider when examining wounds:
  Ensure the entire wound is visible, even if this requires removing or cutting clothing.
  If the injury is to an extremity, do the following:
  o Ensure that the victim is able to move all joints beyond the wound through a complete range of motion.
  o Evaluate the victim's circulation by squeezing the tip of the victim's fingers or toes, with one finger over the nail and another over the pad of the finger, for one second. After releasing, the color should return to the nail bed within two to three seconds. If not, the circulation may be compromised. This test is unreliable in cold weather.
  Proper light for examination is paramount. A headlamp is an excellent hands-free tool to improve visualization in the wilderness.

TYPES OF SKIN WOUNDS

Abrasions

  These "road rash" injuries can range from minor scrapes that involve the superficial layers of the skin to injuries that cause major skin disruption, as seen in high-speed crashes.
  More serious injuries may involve muscle tissue and can be serious enough to require skin grafting.
  Most abrasions result in minimal blood loss but can be very painful due to exposure of many nerve endings.
  These injuries are commonly contaminated and contain foreign objects, such as dirt and rocks, depending on how they occurred.

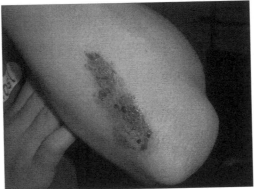

Figure 27.1 Abrasion

Lacerations

  A cut to the skin is called a laceration.
  There are many different types of lacerations:
  □ The laceration may be straight, curved, or even star-shaped ("burst").
  □ Puncture wounds are lacerations with depth greater than length. These have a higher risk of infection and often have foreign objects embedded deeply in the wound. Due to the depth and unknown pathway, puncture wounds are more difficult to examine and clean.
  □ Bites from animals and humans may cause puncture or laceration wounds. Because mouths are full of bacteria, these wounds are at high risk for infection.

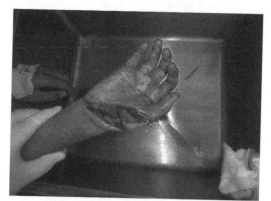

Figure 27.2. Photo courtesy of www.jacknaimsnotes.com

Blisters

Blisters that develop in the wilderness most commonly form due to frictional forces while hiking. Improperly broken-in or poorly fitting shoes are the most common causes.

A blister is typically preceded by a "hot spot," which is a painful red area formed from the frictional forces. Presentation may range from minor and even painless fluid collections to debilitating injuries that may require evacuation. Infection of a blister is the worst complication, although pain and disability are more common.

Burns

There are two important criteria to be considered with burns:
1. The degree of the burn
2. The size of the burn in relation to the victim's total body area

Superficial (First Degree) Burn

The skin is typically reddened, and the victim will likely complain of pain.

A common example of a first-degree burn is sunburn.

While first-degree burns are painful, they are the easiest type of burn to treat and evacuation is generally unnecessary.

Partial Thickness (Second Degree) Burn

The skin will be blistered and either red or possibly pale white to yellow.

Second-degree burns are painful and involve deeper skin damage.

Second-degree burns can be significant, especially if they involve a large area of skin.

Evacuation may be required depending on the extent of the skin (amount of body surface area) involved and the location of the burn.

Full Thickness (Third Degree) Burn

All layers of the skin have been burned, including blood vessels and nerves in the subcutaneous tissue.

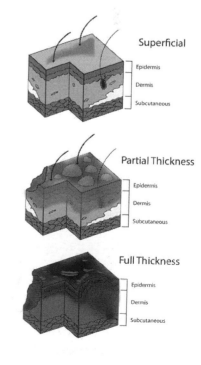

Figure 27.3

The flesh may be charred, but the victim generally feels no pain from a full-thickness burn because the nerve endings have been destroyed.

Painful second-degree burns may surround the third-degree burn.

Burn Size

Burn area should be estimated to help determine the need for evacuation. This can easily be accomplished by using the rule of nines to determine total body surface area (TBSA):

Each arm:	9% TBSA
Each leg:	9% TBSA
Front of trunk:	18% TBSA
Back of trunk:	18% TBSA
Head and neck:	9% TBSA
Groin:	1% TBSA

Another estimation guide is to use the patient's palm, which represents approximately 1% TBSA.

TREATMENT

Control Active Bleeding

First line of action: Direct pressure.

Application of direct pressure controls bleeding from most wounds. Using the cleanest material available, apply direct pressure to the source of bleeding. Larger wounds may require direct pressure for several minutes. Scalp wounds may require continuous direct pressure for up to 30 to 60 minutes. One can apply a pressure dressing over a wound to apply a continuous pressure. This can be performed by holding the primary dressing and wrapping a compressive ("Ace") wrap around the dressing and the extremity or area of concern. Do not place a compressive dressing around the neck in such a way that it would inhibit breathing.

Second line of action: Pressure points and elevation.

If direct pressure does not stop bleeding after about 20 minutes, or if bleeding is brisk and cannot immediately be controlled with pressure, elevate the limb above the heart and apply pressure to the pressure points in the victim's armpit (axillary artery) or groin (femoral artery). Generally, one will do this after placing a pressure dressing on the wound, so it is an additive treatment regimen.

Last resort: Tourniquet. If the first two methods do not stop the bleeding, AND if the victim is in danger of bleeding to death, use a tourniquet.

Tourniquets should typically be used only as a last result. However, if a patient is bleeding extensively from a wound, you must first stop this massive hemorrhage rapidly as a victim can lose most of their blood volume in a matter of minutes with major arterial or venous bleeding. In the wilderness, you cannot replace this blood and the victim may be required to be much more active than the typical hospitalized patient.

- This step is applicable for only major bleeding and does not include injuries with only minor oozing that will be addressed later in the secondary survey. Generally, these types of injuries are rare in the wilderness but can have fatal consequences if not treated rapidly.

- This treatment usually consists of the placement of a tourniquet if it is an extremity injury. If one does not have a tourniquet or if the injury is not amenable to the use of a tourniquet (e.g. facial or torso wound), then a pressure dressing directly on the area of bleeding is the best option.

- The placement of the tourniquet does not mandate that the tourniquet stay in place until the patient reaches definitive medical care. The expectation is that that the rescuer will reassess the wound and the bleeding after the patient has been stabilized in the secondary survey and ongoing assessment stage.

  - ☐ Tourniquets are to be used only if the wound is on an arm or leg.
  - ☐ A tourniquet is a band applied around an arm or leg so tightly that all circulation below the band is cut off. Be aware that if a tourniquet cuts off the blood supply for a sufficient period of time to cause tissue damage from lack of oxygen supply, everything below the tourniquet may require amputation.
  - ☐ To make a tourniquet, take a strip of cloth at least two inches wide. Never use wire, twine, cord, or any other thin material that will cut the skin.
  - ☐ Using an overhand knot, tie the material in a half-knot two inches above to the wound, between the wound and the heart.
  - ☐ Place a stick or rod on top of that half-knot and complete the knot on top of the stick.
  - ☐ Tighten the bandage by turning the stick until the bandage is tight enough to stop the bleeding.
  - ☐ Secure the stick so the tourniquet won't come loose. This may require taping it down.
  - ☐ Write on the victim's forehead the time you applied the tourniquet. This is an obvious note to the health care providers caring for this victim in case you are not able to talk with them directly about the care of that victim.

Irrigation

"High-pressure" irrigation is the most important intervention to prevent infection and to decrease bacterial content for most wounds.

- Irrigate the wound with a forceful stream of disinfected water or saline. This can be created a number of ways:
  - ☐ If available, use a syringe to create a high-pressure stream for irrigation.
  - ☐ Fill a plastic bag or hydration system with the cleanest fluid available (tap water has been shown to protect against infection as effectively as sterile saline). Poke a small hole in a corner of the bag, and then close the top of the bag to create a seal in order to force a stream of water from the bag.
  - ☐ A plastic water bottle with an adjustable top may also be used if a stream can be produced.
- Gently pull apart the wound edges while irrigating. Rinse the wound forcefully with the water, protecting your skin and eyes from fluid splashes. The more fluid used to irrigate the wound, the better. Use at least one liter per wound if water is in sufficient supply.
- Do not forcefully drive water deep into puncture wounds; it can push bacteria and debris further into the surrounding tissue.

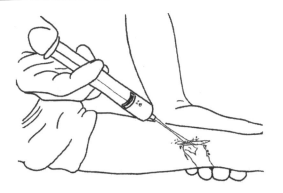

Figure 27.4. Irrigating a Wound

Foreign Matter in Wounds

It is important to remove visible foreign matter from the wound in order to minimize the chance of infection and to prevent skin tattooing. This may be problematic, particularly if one is unable to adequately visualize the entire wound. Once all visible foreign matter is removed from a wound, another round of irrigation should be performed.

Wound Closure

The primary goal of wound closure is to bring the wound edges together in order to improve the functional status of the victim and to minimize the scar that results from the wound.

A common misconception regarding wounds is that closure of the wound decreases the chance of infection. In reality, closure of the wound may increase the chance of infection compared to packing the wound and dressing it properly.

An important consideration is that there is generally no increase in scarring if one packs and dresses a wound and then closes it three to five days later, as opposed to closing it at the time of injury. Packing and dressing a wound with delayed closure is termed *delayed primary closure*. If one is in the wilderness for a period of five days or less, then delayed primary closure is a very good option.

Methods of skin closure that can be utilized in the wilderness that do not involve suturing include the following:

Taping the wound:

The tape should close the wound so the edges of the wound touch (approximate), but not so tightly that the tape squeezes the wound rigidly shut.

If needed, cut away the hair around the edges of the wound with scissors so that the tape will adhere better. Do not shave the area around the wound, as shaving may increase the chance of infection.

Cut the tape into thin strips approximately four to six mm in width.

Place the tape perpendicular to the wound, allowing an adherent length of tape for at least one inch on each side of the wound.

Place the strips of tape approximately two to five millimeters apart.

If micropore tape (medical tape) is not available, then one may use duct tape. However, when using the duct tape, punch holes in duct tape from the sticky side out using a safety pin. This allows fluid to drain from the wound through the tape.

Recently released Dermabond "skin glue" is effective for closing wounds.

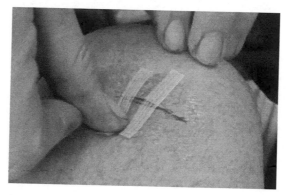

Figure 27.5 Taping a wound - Photo courtesy of Remote Medicine Ireland

Hair-knotting technique to close scalp wounds:

If the hair is at least one inch long on both sides of the wound, it can be tied or glued together to close the wound edges.

Separate the hair on each side of the wound.

On each side of the wound, roll several strands of hair together.

Pull these strands across the wound to the opposite side. Depending upon the length of the rolled strands, these can be tied or twisted to pull the wound edges together. If the hair is twisted together, applying "super glue" so that the hair does not untwist will hold it more securely.

Several groups of rolled strands may be needed to close a long wound.

Dressing

Wound dressing is important for protection from the environment and prevention of infection. This may be accomplished in a number of ways:

If available, apply antibiotic/antiseptic ointment and cover with a sterile, non-stick dressing. Cover this with an absorbent gauze dressing and secure with tape.

If a commercial non-stick pad or dressing is not available, improvise using a gauze pad and antibiotic/antiseptic ointment. Cover this dressing with an absorbent gauze dressing, then secure with tape.

If the injury is on a flexible part of the body – an elbow or a finger, for example – immobilize the joint with a splint to prevent reopening of the wound.

Dressing changes and wound checks should be performed at least once daily in the wilderness. Most infections begin within 48 hours, but aggressive and gas-forming infections may begin within hours.

Topical Antibiotics/Antiseptics

Topical antibiotic/antiseptic ointments are appropriate for all skin wounds.

Ointments can be obtained over the counter. There is no best ointment, although allergic reactions may be more common if neomycin is a component.

Another topical antimicrobial is honey. The natural compounds in unprocessed honey make it an effective, inexpensive and readily available alternative to ointment.

TYPES OF WOUNDS

Abrasions

Abrasions should be irrigated as described above.

In addition to irrigation, abrasions that are very dirty may require vigorous scrubbing in order to remove the embedded dirt and other foreign material. Although scrubbing is painful, it is important to ensure proper healing with minimization of infection and tattooing from retained foreign matter.

Dress and treat as indicated above.

Amputations

Once bleeding has been controlled, determine if the amputated part is large enough to be re-implanted.

Candidates for re-implantation include:

- ☐ Thumb amputation
- ☐ Multiple finger amputation
- ☐ Single finger amputation below (toward the knuckle) the joint directly adjacent to the nail bed
- ☐ Injuries in children

The amputated part should ideally be soaked in sterile gauze and then placed in a bag. The bag is then transported on ice with the victim to definitive care as soon as possible. Do <u>not</u> place the amputated part directly on the ice, as this could cause a freezing injury.

Lacerations

Most lacerations can be treated as described under General Considerations above. Special considerations include the following:

Scalp Lacerations

The extent and severity of scalp lacerations are often initially obscured by surrounding hair that is matted with blood.

Copious irrigation is often necessary to visualize the laceration.

Hair may be trimmed if necessary, but this should be limited to the immediate area of the laceration, since the surrounding hair can later be twisted into strands and used to approximate the wound edges.

Facial Lacerations

Superficial lacerations to the face may be managed in the wilderness. However, those involving the eyelids or the ears or those with deep injuries require evacuation.

As with other lacerations, high-pressure irrigation is the method of choice for mechanical cleaning.

Deep Lacerations to the Arm, Hand, or Foot

Management of deep extremity lacerations in the wilderness requires careful judgment because of the potential involvement of underlying structures.

This is especially true with the hand, where critical structures lie perilously close to the surface.

Therefore, a detailed evaluation of all wounds to the arms, hands, and feet should be performed, including these steps:

☐ Test the strength of the extremity beyond the wound because tendon injuries may not be obvious at initial evaluation.

☐ Evaluate the base of the wound through full range of motion of the extremity because tendon lacerations may easily be missed if examined in just one position.

☐ Check sensation beyond the wound. This is easily accomplished by asking the victim to compare sensation beyond the wound with sensation at the same location on the uninvolved arm, hand, leg, or foot.

Any evidence of loss of movement, circulation, or sensation beyond a wound mandates evacuation.

Puncture Wounds

Puncture wounds should NOT be forcefully irrigated because this may further push in bacteria, dirt and debris. Instead, the surface should be thoroughly scrubbed, and the wound should be dressed as indicated above, without attempts at closure.

Puncture wounds should be reevaluated more frequently than are simple lacerations, as they are at higher risk for infection.

Bites

Bites should be cleaned extensively, examined closely for foreign objects, such as teeth, and dressed as described.

Bites are at higher risk for infection due to bacterial contamination from mouth germs and therefore should be checked regularly.

Blisters

If a small blister or hot spot forms, protect the area by cutting a hole the size of the blister in a piece of moleskin. Secure the moleskin around the blister to act as a shield to the area. Anchor the moleskin with benzoin or a similar product, and secure with tape. Build up several layers of moleskin or mole foam if necessary. Do not open or puncture small blisters.

Studies have shown the effectiveness of dual layer blist-o-ban in preventing and treating blisters.

If the blister is large (quarter-sized) or ruptured, wash the area and puncture the base of the blister with a sterile needle or safety pin. Carefully remove the external flap of skin from the blister, and apply an antibiotic/antiseptic ointment, covering the blister with a sterile dressing. This can be protected with moleskin or mole foam.

Inspect daily for signs of infection. If an intact blister appears infected, drain it by removing the external flap and seek medical attention.

Burns

Superficial Burns (First-Degree Burns)

- [ ] Treat first-degree burns with aloe-vera gel.
- [ ] For comfort, cool the area with damp wet cloths.
- [ ] Silvadene cream can be used.

Partial-Thickness and Full-Thickness Burns

- [ ] Gently clean the burn with cool water and remove loose skin and debris.
- [ ] Trim away all loose skin with scissors.
- [ ] Blisters larger than the size of a quarter, those that are leaking, or those that will obviously burst because of rough handling, may be drained and the flap removed carefully.
- [ ] Apply a thin layer of Silvadene or other antimicrobial ointment to the burn and cover with a non-adhering, sterile dressing. Change the dressing at least twice daily.
- [ ] Do not apply ice to burns for more than 15 minutes, as this will cause more damage due to a potential frostbite injury.

Signs of Infection

These symptoms indicate that the skin is infected:
- [ ] Pain that is worse than it was at the time of the initial insult
- [ ] Redness around the wound edges that is spreading out from the wound (commonly, there is mild redness/pinkness right at the wound edge)
- [ ] Red streaking away from the wound, particularly towards the heart
- [ ] Swelling of the wound and the surrounding area
- [ ] Purulent drainage (pus) from the wound
- [ ] Swollen lymph nodes in the armpit for arm/hand injuries or the groin for leg/foot injuries
- [ ] Fever

PREVENTION

Because skin injuries are among the most common ailments in the wilderness, simple preventive measures can be taken to decrease their incidence.

- [ ] Wear gloves when working with objects that can cause you to scrape your hand or develop blisters.
- [ ] Alcohol and drug use is a significant risk factor for developing wounds in the backcountry. Their use should be kept to a minimum in the backcountry and entirely prohibited around risky activities.
- [ ] Improper knife handling is responsible for an excessive number of preventable skin injuries.
- [ ] Adequate lighting should be used to avoid falls and other injuries.
- [ ] Tetanus is a life-threatening infection, and many wounds in the wilderness are considered tetanus-prone. ALL individuals should have their tetanus immunization updated before participating in wilderness activities.

EVACUATION GUIDLINES

Victims who have wounds with the following characteristics should be considered for evacuation:
- Complex or mutilating wounds
- Grossly contaminated with penetrating debris
- Lacerations of the ear, eyelid, or cartilage
- Penetration of bone, joint, or tendon
- Bites of the hands, legs, or feet
- Amputations

Wounds with signs of serious or progressive infection should be evacuated as soon as possible.

Burn evacuation guidelines include:
- Partial-thickness burns greater than 10% body surface area
- Full-thickness burns greater than 1% body surface area
- Partial- or full-thickness burns involving the face, hands, feet or genitals
- Electrical burns
- If the burn victim is medically ill
- Burns complicated by smoke or heat inhalation (evidence of smoke inhalation include difficulty breathing, hoarse voice, singed nasal hairs, or carbon in patient's sputum)

QUESTIONS

1. **What is the most important intervention to help prevent infection of a wound?**
   a) Antibiotic/antiseptic ointment
   b) High-pressure irrigation
   c) A sterile wound dressing
   d) Removal of very small foreign objects from the wound

2. **Which burn does NOT require evacuation?**
   a) A camper wakes up when his tent has caught on fire because he did not properly put out his campfire. He is able to evacuate from the tent, but is coughing frequently, complains of shortness of breath, and has singed nose hairs.
   b) A victim with burns on the forearm after attempting to treat a snakebite by placing jumper cables adjacent to the area and starting his car.
   c) A victim with four centimeters of redness on the back of the forearm after brushing against hot firewood.
   d) A victim with burns and blistering to the bottom of his foot after stepping on hot coals.

3. **Which of the following is necessary to evaluate when examining a wound in the wilderness?**
   a) Location, extent, and depth of the wound
   b) Presence or absence of dirt, debris, or foreign objects
   c) Bone, tendon, or joint involvement
   d) Sensation and circulation beyond the wound
   e) All of the above

4. **Which wound requires evacuation?**
   a) A six cm laceration of the head secured by tying strands of hair together
   b) A puncture wound of the foot that has developed surrounding redness, has pus draining from it, and is extremely painful upon which to walk
   c) A three-day-old two cm arm laceration that has some redness around it without pus or worsening pain
   d) A four cm leg laceration that has been irrigated, has no foreign body, bone, tendon, or joint involvement, and is secured with tape

5. **Which is the best way to treat a simple friction blister the size of a dime?**
   a) Clean the area, place a ring of moleskin over it, and cover it with athletic tape
   b) Ignore it; most blisters rupture or stop hurting sooner or later
   c) Puncture with a needle, remove the flap, and cover with athletic tape
   d) Place a ring of moleskin over the blister, cover everything with tape, and evacuate the victim for antibiotics
   e) Evacuate all friction blisters without treatment in the wilderness

6. **For which of the following wounds should the use of a tourniquet be considered?**
   a) An amputation of half of the little finger
   b) An amputation of the leg at the level of the knee, sustained in a high-speed four-wheeler collision, with bleeding mostly controlled by direct pressure and pressure points
   c) A rapidly bleeding scalp laceration that continues despite 30 minutes of pressure
   d) An artery laceration at the elbow due to an open fracture from a 15-foot fall that continues to bleed despite 30 minutes of direct pressure and use of pressure points

7. **What is the best way to transport amputated digits?**
   a) In milk
   b) In the mouth
   c) In the victim's pocket
   d) Wrapped in sterile water-soaked gauze, placed in a bag and transported on ice
   e) Placed directly on ice and then placed in a plastic bag

8. **Which best describes a partial-thickness burn?**
   a) A large burn with exposed muscle and bone
   b) A painful area of redness without blistering or tissue loss
   c) A painful area of redness with blistering
   d) A burn that has a central painless white area

ANSWERS
1. b 2. c 3. e 4. b 5. a 6. d 7. d 8. c

Acronyms

Potential Sources of Major Bleeding

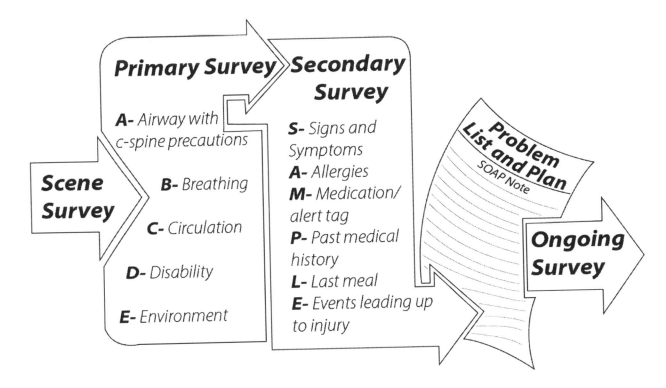

CHEST	The chest is a common source of bleeding, particularly in high-energy trauma. Look for shortness of breath, pain with breathing, and coughing up blood. Examine for chest tenderness, crepitance over the ribs and sternum, flail chest and crackling noises of the chest consistent with air under the skin.
ABDOMEN/PELVIS	Assume abdominal and/or pelvis bleeding in every trauma victim until proven otherwise. Look for bruising over the abdomen and pelvis. Palpate for abdominal and pelvic tenderness on compression.
RENAL	Usually the bleeding is from the kidneys. Look for blood in the urine if you have a prolonged time with the victim. Examine for tenderness of the spine and chest and the lowest level of the ribs.

THIGH	This may occur if there is a femur fracture. Look for deformity, swelling and bruising of the thigh. Palpate for tenderness and crepitance of the thigh.
SKIN/STREET	This is the most obvious place for a rescuer to detect blood. A common error in the wilderness setting is the failure to remove clothing or to roll the patient to look for bleeding. Also, ensure that you survey the area immediately surrounding the victim for a large amount of blood on the ground that may have come from the victim. Specifically an arterial injury that bleeds significantly may be in spasm at the time you are evaluating the victim and not be an obvious source of bleeding.

Secondary Survey: Characterizing the Pain

O   Onset: When did the pain start?
P   Provokes/Palliates: What makes the pain better or worse?
Q   Quality: What does the pain feel like?
R   Radiation: Does the pain move anywhere?
S   Severity: How bad is the pain on a scale of 1 – 10?
T   Time: How long has the pain been going on? When did it start?

Primary Survey: Disability
Level of Responsiveness

A   Alert
V   Verbal – Awakens briefly, withdraws, or moans when spoken to
P   Pain – Awakens briefly, withdraws, or moans in response to painful stimuli
U   Unresponsive – No response to any stimuli

Criteria for "clearing" a C-Spine

C   Cervical midline tenderness
S   Sensory-motor deficit (numbness/weakness)
P   Pain or psychological distractor
I   Intoxication
N   Neurologic deficit (loss of alertness)
E   Events (sufficient mechanism to cause neck injury)

Glossary of Terms

A

abandonment: To leave a patient in need of medical attention alone or with someone who is not capable of providing care.

abduction: Movement away from the midline of the body.

abrasion: A type of wound that consists of one or more layers of skin being scraped away.

acclimatization: The process of physiologically adjusting to a new environment, such as a higher altitude.

Achilles tendon: The tendon that connects the muscles of the lower leg to the heel bone.

acidosis: A condition that is produced by the build up of acid or the reduction of base in the body.

ACL: See **anterior cruciate ligament.**

acute: An immediate problem that is not chronic.

acute mountain sickness (AMS): Nonspecific problems caused by the inability to acclimatize to higher altitudes; the first stage in a progression that can lead to **high-altitude cerebral edema.**

adduction: Movement toward the midline of the body.

AED: Shorthand for automated external defibrillator.

AGE: See **arterial gas embolism.**

alkalosis: A condition produced by the accumulation of base or the reduction of acid in the body.

allergen: Any substance that causes an allergic reaction.

AWLS: Shorthand for Advanced Wilderness Life Support.

alveoli: Microscopic sacs of the lungs where gas exchange takes place.

ambulatory: Able to walk.

amenorrhea: The suppression or unusual absence of menstruation.

AMI: Acute myocardial infarction; a sudden heart attack.

amnesia: Loss of memory.

amniotic sack: The thin membrane that covers the fetus and placenta, containing amniotic fluid.

amputation:	To cut off a limb or other appendage of the body, especially in a surgical operation.
AMS:	See **acute mountain sickness.**
analgesic:	A medication that alleviates pain without loss of consciousness.
anaphylaxis:	A sudden severe and potentially fatal allergic reaction in somebody sensitive to a substance, marked by a drop in blood pressure, difficulty in breathing, itching, and swelling.
anesthetic:	An agent that produces a partial or complete loss of sensation.
aneurysm:	Abnormal bulging of a blood vessel, usually in an artery.
angina pectoris:	A medical condition in which lack of blood to the heart causes severe chest pains.
anterior:	Front surface.
anterior cruciate ligament (ACL):	One of the two ligaments that cross within the knee.
antibiotic:	A substance that prevents growth of or destroys microorganisms.
anticholinergic:	An agent that blocks nerve impulses which are part of the stress response.
antidiarrheal:	A substance that is used to prevent and treat diarrhea.
anti-emetic:	A substance that is used to prevent and treat vomiting.
antihistamine:	A drug that is used to counteract the effects of histamines.
anti-inflammatory:	A substance used to reduce inflammation.
antipyretic:	An agent that reduces or alleviates a fever.
antiseptic:	An agent that reduces or prevents infection, especially by eliminating or reducing the growth of microorganisms that cause disease or decay.
antivenin:	An antiserum containing antibodies to a specific venom – same thing as antivenom.
antivenom:	An antiserum containing antibodies to a specific venom – same thing as antivenin.
aorta:	The main artery that carries blood from the left ventricle of the heart travels to the body.
aortic valve:	The valve between the left ventricle and the aorta.
apnea:	A temporary suspension or absence of breathing.
appendicitis:	Inflammation of the appendix, causing severe pain.
aqueous humor:	Salty liquid that fills the cornea.
arachnoid:	The middle of the three membranes that envelop the brain and spinal cord
arterial gas embolism (AGE):	An air bubble present in the arterial blood stream.
arteriole:	Small artery.
arteriosclerosis:	Hardening, Thickening, and loss of elasticity of the arteries.
artery:	A vessel that carries blood from the heart to the rest of the body.
asphyxia:	A condition caused by an insufficient intake of oxygen.
asthma:	A disease of the respiratory system characterized by shortness of breath and wheezing due to swelling of bronchi and their mucous membranes.

asystole:	Absence of the heartbeat and all other activity in the heart.
ATA:	Atmosphere absolute; the pressure of the earths atmosphere.
ataxia:	Loss of muscle coordination leading to trouble in maintaining balance.
atherosclerosis:	Obstruction of the blood flow due to clogging of the arteries from fatty deposits and other debris.
atrium:	The upper chamber of each half of the heart that takes blood from the veins and pumps it into a ventricle.
auscultate:	Listen.
AVPU scale:	For *Alert, Verbal, Pain, Unresponsive*—a scale for measuring a patient's level of consciousness.
avulsion:	The tearing away or separation of part of the body, usually includes a piece of skin left hanging as a flap.
AWLS:	Advanced Wilderness Life Support

B

bacteria:	Single-cell microorganisms.
baroreceptors:	Pressure-sensitive nerve ending.
barosinusitis:	Pain or inflammation of nasal sinuses as a result of pressure changes; also known as middle ear squeeze.
barotitis:	Inflammation of the ear as a result of changes in pressure.
barotitis media:	Inflammation of the middle ear as a result of changes in pressure; also known as middle ear squeeze.
barotrauma:	An injury that is caused by a change in pressure, as in scuba diving.
basal metabolic rate (BMR):	The constant rate at which a human body consumes energy to drive chemical reactions and generate heat to maintain a sufficient core temperature at rest.
Battle's sign:	Bruising behind and below the ears, which indicates a fracture to the base of the skull.
bipolar disease:	Cyclical pattern of shifts between depression and mania.
bleb:	Fluid-filled blister.
blood pressure:	The pressure exerted by circulating blood against the walls of the arteries.
BWLS:	Basic Wilderness Life Support.
BMR:	See **basal metabolic rate.**
bony crepitus:	Sound or feel of broken bone ends grinding against one another.
BP:	See **blood pressure.**
bradycardia:	Slowness of heart rate.
brain stem:	Part of the brain that connects the cerebral hemispheres to the spinal cord.
breech presentation:	A birth when the baby emerges feet or buttocks first.
bronchiole:	A small airway of the lung.

bronchitis:	Inflammation of the mucous membranes of the bronchi causing breathing problems and severe coughing.
bronchospasm:	Spasms that take place in the muscles of the bronchi.
bronchus:	One of the two large airways branching off from the trachea which carries air to the lungs.
BVM:	Bag valve mask. A patient ventilation device.

C

capillary:	A narrow thin-walled blood vessel where gas exchange occurs between the bloodstream and the tissues.
cardiac arrest:	The termination of heart muscle activity.
cardiogenic:	Originating in the heart.
cardiopulmonary resuscitation (CPR):	Artificial respirations and manual chest compressions that help stimulate lung and heart activity.
cardiovascular system:	The heart, the blood vessels, and the blood.
carotid artery:	A large artery on each side of the neck that supplies blood to the head.
cartilage:	Strong, elastic tissue in the body that forms protective pads where bone meets bone.
catheter:	A tube that is inserted into the body in order to remove or insert fluids.
centruroides:	A particularly potent species of scorpion commonly found in Arizona.
cerebellum:	The part of the brain that helps control balance and movement.
cerebral:	In relation to the cerebrum.
cerebrospinal fluid (CSF):	The fluid that surrounds the brain and spinal cord.
cerebrovascular accident (CVA):	Interruption of regular blood flow to a part of the brain which results in a stroke.
cerebrum:	The largest, frontal part of the brain that consists of two symmetrical hemispheres.
cervical vertebrae:	The first seven bones pertaining to the spinal column; the neck bones.
cervix:	The narrow opening at the lower end of the uterus.
CHF:	See **congestive heart failure.**
Chief complaint:	The principal complaint of a patient. Also CC.
chronic obstructive pulmonary disease (COPD):	A collection of diseases sharing the common symptoms of airway obstruction in the small to medium airways, excessive secretions, and/or constriction of the bronchial tubes.
chronic:	A condition of slow progression or long duration; not acute.
clavicle:	Collarbone.
closed pneumothorax:	A tear in the lining of the lung that results in air gathering in the pleural space with no open wounds.
CNS:	For *Central Nervous System*. The brain and spinal cord.
CO:	Carbon monoxide.

coccyx:	The triangular bone at the base of the spinal column, consisting of four fused vertebra; the tailbone.
cochlea:	Cone-shaped tube situated in the inner ear.
coma:	An prolonged state of deep unconsciousness from which the patient cannot be awakened.
comminuted fracture:	A fracture where the bone is crushed or splintered.
conduction:	Heat that is lost from a warmer object when it comes in contact with a colder object.
congestive heart failure (CHF):	A condition in which blood and tissue fluids congest due to the insufficiency of the heart.
conjunctiva:	The delicate membrane lining the eyes.
constipation:	Infrequent or difficult bowel movements where the feces are hard and dry.
contusion:	A bruise.
convection:	Heat lost directly into air or water caused by movement.
COPD:	See **chronic obstructive pulmonary disease.**
coronary artery:	The vessel that supplies blood to the heart muscle.
cruciate ligament:	One of the crossed ligaments that holds the knee joint together. The anterior cruciate ligament is attached to the rear of the femur and the front of the tibia; the posterior cruciate ligament is attached to the front of the femur and the rear of the tibia.
cryptosporidium:	Protozoa that is found in surface waters.
CSF:	See **cerebrospinal fluid.**
CSM:	For *Circulation, Sensation, Motion.*
CVA:	See **cerebrovascular accident.**
cyanosis:	A condition in which the skin and mucous membranes take on a bluish color because there is not enough oxygen in the blood.

D

DAN:	For *Divers Alert Network.*
DCS:	See **decompression sickness.**
decompression sickness (DCS):	A divers condition characterized by buildup of nitrogen bubbles in tissues after breathing compressed air and ascending too quickly.
DEET:	An insect repellent.
defibrillation:	To stop fibrillation of the heart by using electricity or drugs.
dentin:	The calcified area of a tooth surrounding the **pulp**.
dermatitis:	Skin inflammation.
diabetes mellitus:	A disease in which the pancreas produces an insufficient amount of insulin or the cells of the body are unresponsive to insulin. Blood sugars are high.
diaphoresis:	Profuse sweating.
diarrhea:	frequent passage of unformed, watery bowel movement.

diastolic pressure/dias-tole: Pressure exerted by blood on the walls of arteries throughout the relaxation phase of the heart activity.

dislocation: The displacement of a body part, especially of a bone from its usual fitting in a joint.

distal: Away from the center.

distal interphalageal joint: The distal joint of the finger; also known as the DIP joint.

diuretic: A substance that causes increased flow of urine.

ductus deferens: Excretory duct of the testicle.

dura mater: The tough outermost membrane of the **meninges,** covering the brain and spinal cord.

dysentery: A disease caused by infection of bacteria, marked by severe bacteria that may produce blood and mucus in the stool.

dysmenorrhea: Severe pain associated with menstruation.

dyspnea: Difficulty in breathing.

E

ecchymosis: Bruising.

ectopic pregnancy: A pregnancy in which the developing fetus implants outside of the womb, usually in a fallopian tube.

edema: Swelling that is caused caused by a buildup of excess fluid.

efface: Thin, as in the cervix during childbirth.

electromagnetic spec-trum: The complete range of electromagnetic radiation from the shortest waves gamma rays to the longest radio waves.

embolism: Obstruction of a blood vessel by a clot of blood, a gas bubble, or a foreign substance.

emetics: Causing vomiting.

emesis: Vomit.

emphysema: Chronic pulmonary disease characterized by destruction of the alveoli.

enamel: Hard layer that covers and protects the crown of a tooth.

endometrium: The mucous membrane that lines the uterus.

envenomation: Poisoning from a venomous bite or sting.

epidermis: The thin outermost layer of the skin.

epididymis: The organ situated behind the testicle that stores sperm.

epidural: Located above the dura meter.

epigastric: The upper part of the abdomen.

epiglottis: The structure overlying the larynx which helps to prevent food or liquid from entering the windpipe during swallowing.

epistaxis: Nosebleed.

eschar: Scar.

esophagus:	The passage down which food moves between the throat and the stomach.
ETOH:	Alcohol.
eustachian tube:	The tube that extends from the middle ear to the back of the throat.
evaporation:	A process in which something is changed from a liquid to a vapor.
eversion:	A condition of being turned outwards.
evisceration:	A condition in which abdominal contents are exposed and protruding out from an open wound.
exhalation:	The act of breathing out.

F

fallopian tube:	The tube that extends from the ovary to the uterus.
fascia:	A sheet or band of connective tissue covering or binding together parts of the body such as muscles.
febrile:	Relating to a fever.
femoral:	Relating to the femur.
fibula:	Small lower leg bone between the knee and ankle.
fimbria:	Small, fingerlike constructions found at the end of the **fallopian tube.**
flail chest:	A condition where multiple ribs are fractured in two or more places, creating a floating section of rib.
fracture:	A break in a bone.
frostbite:	Localized tissue damage caused by prolonged exposure to freezing conditions.
frostnip:	Superficial frostbite.
fungus:	A primitive life form that reproduces by spores and lives by absorbing nutrients from organic matter.
fx:	Shorthand for *fracture.*

G

gallstone:	A small hard mass that forms in the gallbladder, sometimes as a result of infection or blockage.
gastric distension:	A condition that occurs as a result of air overinflating the stomach.
gastritis:	Inflammation of the stomach lining.
gastroenteritis:	Stomach and intestinal inflammation.
germ:	A microorganism, especially one that can cause disease.
Giardia Iamblia:	Protozoa with flagella found in surface water.
gingiva:	The gum around the roots of the teeth.
glottis:	The long opening of the vocal cords and space between them at the trachea.
glucagon:	A hormone that raises the concentration of glucose in the blood.
gluteals:	Buttock muscles.

greenstick fracture: A fracture that only extends part way through the bone, usually occurring in children.

grief: Great sadness, especially as a result of a loss.

gross negligence: Severe deviation from the standard of care.

guarding: To protect an injured area through muscle tension and/or physical positioning.

H

HACE: See **high-altitude cerebral edema.**

hamstring: A muscle in the back of the upper leg behind the knee.

HAPE: See **high-altitude pulmonary edema.**

heat cramps: Painful spasm of major muscles that are being exercised; caused by dehydration in association with electrolyte depletion.

heat exhaustion: Weakness produced by fluid loss from excessive sweating in a hot environment that causes compensatory shock.

heatstroke: a condition caused by prolonged exposure to high temperatures, in which people experience high fever, headaches, hot dry skin, physical exhaustion, and sometimes physical collapse and coma.

helminth: A parasitic worm.

hematemesis: The presence of blood in the vomit.

hematoma: Pooling of blood in the form of a tumor.

hematuria: The presence of blood in the urine.

hemoptysis: Coughing up of blood.

hemorrhage: Bleeding.

hemostasis: Control of blood flow.

hemothorax: Blood in the pleural space.

high-altitude cerebral edema (HACE):   A condition in which fluid collects in the patient's brain as a result of extremes of elevation gain.

high-altitude pulmonary edema (HAPE):   A condition when fluid moves from the pulmonary capillaries and fills the alveolar spaces in response to extreme elevation gain.

histamine: A natural substance released by the immune system in the body which responds to an injury or foreign protein.

humerus: Upper arm bone.

hx: Shorthand for *history*.

I

IM: For *Intramuscular*.

immersion foot: An injury that causes inadequate circulation and tissue damage which occurs as a result of prolonged contact with cold and often moisture.

immersion syndrome: The immediate death which follows immersion in cold water.

implied consent: When a patient is unconscious, a minor (if a parent or guardian is unavailable to give consent), or for any other reason unable to decide to be treated, it can be legally assumed that he or she would desire treatment if he or she were capable of making the decision.

incision: A smooth-edged cut made in the skin by a sharp edge.

incontinence: The loss of bladder and/or bowel control.

inferior: Below.

inferior vena cava: The large vein carrying blood from the abdomen, pelvis, and lower limbs to the heart.

inflammation: Localized changes in tissue size, color, and temperature, as a reaction to injury.

informed consent: The decision a patient makes to be treated after having been informed of the benefits and potential risks of the proposed treatment.

inguinal hernia: The most common type of hernia in males which occurs in the region of the groin.

inhalation: Breathing in.

insomnia: Inability to sleep.

insulin: The hormone produced in the pancreas required to regulate the amount of glucose in the bloodstream.

interstitial space: The fluid filled areas between cells.

inversion: Turned inward.

ischemia: Inadequate blood supply to an organ.

IV: For *Intravenous*

J

joint: Where two bones are joined.

K

kidney stone: A hard mass formed in the kidneys and excreted through the urinary tract.

L

laceration: A jagged or torn wound in the skin.

lacrimal: Of or relating to tears.

laryngospasm: A closure of the larynx caused by a spasm which blocks the passage of air to the lungs.

larynx: The structure of cartilage that forms an air passage to the lungs and holds the vocal cords; the "voice box."

lateral: Further from the midline of the body; the outer portion.

lateral collateral ligament: The outside ligament that provides strength and support to the knee.

lesion: A region of an organ or tissue that has been damaged or injured.

ligament: Connective tissue that holds bones together.

lumbar vertebrae: Five bones found in the lower spine between the thoracic vertebrae and the sacrum.

lymphangitis: Inflammation of the walls of the lymph channels or vessels.

M

malaise: A general feeling of discomfort or illness whose exact cause is difficult to diagnose.

malleolus: Rounded protruding end of the tibia or fibula found on either side of the ankle.

mania: A mood disorder marked by periods of great excitement, agitation, accelerated speaking, and hyperactivity.

medial: Closer to the midline of the body; the inner portion.

medial collateral ligament: The inside/inner ligament that is critical to stabilize the knee.

mediastinum: A membrane that separates parts of the body cavity or an organ.

305

meninges: The three membranes – the dura mater, the arachnoid, and the pia mater – that enclose the brain and spinal cord.

meniscus: A crescent-shaped fibrocartilage found in the knee.

metacarpophalangeal joint (MCP): The first joint on the thumb that connects it to the hand.

MI: See **myocardial infarction.**

miscarriage: Expulsion of the fetus from the womb before it can survive.

mitochondria: Intracellular organelles where energy takes place.

mitral valve: The valve located between the left atrium and the left ventricle of the heart.

mittelschmerz: Pain in the area of the ovary associated with ovulation.

MOI: For *Mechanism Of Injury.*

mucus: Slimy fluid secreted by the mucous membranes for lubrication and protection.

myocardial infarction: Death of a portion of the heart muscle resulting from an obstruction of the blood supply to the heart; a heart attack.

myocardium: Heart muscle.

N

nasopharynx: Posterior part of the nose; the part of the pharynx which connects to the nasal cavity above the soft palate.

necrosis: The death of tissue.

negligence: Failure to use proper care that harms another person to whom you owe a duty of care.

neurogenic: Originating in the nervous system.

nitrogen narcosis: A drowsy state caused by an increased concentration of nitrogen gas in body tissues from scuba diving.

NSAID: For *Nonsteroidal anti-inflammatory drug.* A drug administered for inflammation, fever, and pain.

O

oblique fracture: A fracture in which the break runs diagonally across the bone.

odontoid process: A small tooth-like projection of the second cervical vertebra upon which the first cervical vertebra rotates.

olecranon: The bony process of the elbow, on the proximal end of the ulna.

OPA: For *Oropharyngeal airway*. An airway adjunct used in the mouth and throat to aid respiration.

open fracture: A fracture over which the skin is torn or cut.

open pneumothorax: An accumulation of air in the pleural space resulting from a tear in the lining of the lung caused by an open wound.

ophthalmic: Of or relating to the eye.

oropharynx: The back of the mouth; the part of the pharynx between the soft palate and the hyoid bone.

orthopnea: A condition in which it is difficult to breathe while lying down.

orthostatic changes: Increase in heart rate, dizziness, and/or increase in blood pressure caused by sitting or standing from a supine position.

otitis externa: Swelling of the outer ear; "swimmer's ear."

otitis media: Swelling of the middle ear.

ovary: A female reproductive organ in which eggs are produced.

ovulation: The release of an egg from the ovary.

ovum: The egg produced in the ovary.

P

palliate: To soothe pain or make feel better.

palpate: To examine by feeling.

paradoxical respiration: Asymmetrical chest wall movement seen with a **flail chest**.

parasite: An organism that lives in or on another organism.

paresthesia: Loss of feeling or unusual sensations; "pins and needles."

parietal pleura: The portion of the **pleura** that lines the inner chest walls.

patella: The kneecap.

patent:	Clear and unobstructed, as in an airway.
pathogen:	A microorganism which produces disease.
pathological:	Concerning mental or physical disease.
PCL:	See **posterior cruciate ligament.**
PE:	See **pulmonary embolism.**
pedal:	Of or relating to the foot.
pelvic inflammatory disease (PID):	Inflammation of the female genital tract.
perfusion:	The pumping of liquid, typically oxygenated blood, through an organ or tissue.
pericardial sac:	The sac that surrounds the heart.
pericardial tamponade:	Emergency condition in which the pericardial sac is filled with fluid.
perineal:	Region between the anus and vagina or scrotum.
periodontal abscess:	An area characterized by infection and pus formation on the gum.
peripheral:	Of, relating to, or situated near the edge, away from the center.
peripheral nervous system (PNS):	The network of nerves outside the brain and spinal cord.
peritonitis:	Inflammation of the lining of the abdomen (peritoneum).
permethrin:	Insect repellent spray applied to clothing primarily to prevent disease; an insecticide.
PERRL:	For *Pupils Equal Round and Reactive to Light.*
PFD:	For *Personal flotation device.*
phalanges:	Bones located in the fingers or toes.
pia mater:	The inner membrane of the **meninges** in which the brain and spinal cord are surrounded.
placenta:	The organ that nourishes the fetus.
plague:	An epidemic disease caused by the bacteria *Yersinia pestis.*
pleura:	The membrane which lines the chest cavity and in which both lungs are surrounded.
pleural space:	The small potential space between the parietal and visceral layers of the **pleura.**
PMS:	See **premenstrual syndrome.**
pneumonia:	Lung infection or inflammation caused by bacterial or viral infection.
pneumothorax:	An accumulation of air in the pleural space caused by a tear in the lining of the lung.
polyuria:	Excessive production or passage of urine.
posterior:	Back surface.
posterior cruciate ligament (PCL):	One of two ligaments that cross within the knee offering stability.
postictal:	Pertaining to the period following a seizure.

premenstrual syndrome (PMS): Symptoms that occur prior to menstruation.

prolapsed cord: Emergency situation in which the umbilical cord appears in the vaginal canal prior to the baby.

prone: The face-down position.

prostatitis: Inflammation of the prostate.

proximal: Towards the midline of the body; nearest the center.

proximal interphalangeal (PIP) joint: The proximal joint of the finger.

psychogenic: Of a psychological origin or cause.

pulmonary edema: Fluid accumulation in the lungs.

pulmonary embolism: Obstruction of blood flow in a pulmonary artery or arteriole.

pulmonary overinflation syndrome: The condition in which the gas in the lungs over-expands caused by too rapid an ascent when scuba diving.

pulmonary valve: The valve located between the right ventricle and the pulmonary artery.

pulp: The soft portion of the center of a tooth where the nerves and blood vessels are found.

pulpitis: Inflammation of pulp.

pulse pressure: The difference between **systolic pressure** and **diastolic pressure**

puncture: A wound made by the piercing of a pointed object such as knife, bullet, or ice ax.

Q

quadriceps: Thigh muscles used to extend the leg.

quadriplegia: Paralysis of all four appendages.

R

rabies: A contagious and fatal viral infection of the central nervous system transmitted by the bite of an infected mammal.

raccoon eyes: Bruising around the eyes that suggest a skull fracture.

radial: Of or pertaining to the **radius**.

radiation: Heat transmitted by a warm object.

radius: The shorter lower bone in the arm.

reduction: A return to normal anatomical relationship.

respiratory arrest: Cessation of normal breathing.

rhinoviruses: A group of viruses that cause the common cold.

rigor mortis: Stiffness that occurs in a dead body.

RLQ: For *Right Lower Quadrant* of the abdomen.

root: The portion of a tooth beneath the gum.

rotator cuff:	The muscles (supraspinal, infraspinatus, subscapulars, and teres minor) that hold the head of the humerus in the shoulder socket and control rotation of the shoulder.

S

sacrum:	The five fused bones of vertebrae at the bottom of the spine; one of three bones of the pelvic ring.
SAMPLE:	For *Symptoms, Allergies, Medications, Pertinent medical history, Last intake/output, Events.*
scapula:	Shoulder blade.
sclera:	The fibrous tissue that covers the white portion of the eye.
scrotum:	The sac containing the testicles and other parts
of the male reproductive system.	
SCTM:	For *Skin Color, Temperature, Moisture.*
scuba:	For *Self-contained underwater breathing apparatus.*
seizure:	A sudden, abnormal electrical discharge in the brain resulting in altered consciousness.
separation:	Expansion of the spaces between bones.
sepsis:	An illness caused by a buildup of toxins and microorganisms in the blood.
septicemia:	"Blood poisoning" from too much bacteria or their toxins in the blood.
serum:	The watery portion of blood.
shin:	The front of the leg below the knee.
shin splints:	Persistent pain in the shin area caused by repeated impact such as prolonged running.
sinusitis:	Infection of the sinuses.
SOAP:	For *Subjective, Objective, Assessment, Plan.*
sphygmomanometer:	A blood pressure cuff.
spirochete:	A flexible spiral-shaped bacterial microorganism.
spontaneous pneumothorax:	An accumulation of air in the pleural space cased by a tear in the lining of the lung that occurs without trauma.
sprain:	A joint injury in which ligaments are stretched or torn.
sputum:	A mixture of saliva and mucus coughed up from the airway.
sternum:	The breastbone found in the center of the chest.
stoma:	A small artificial opening surgically inserted in the trachea to assist breathing.
strain:	Stretching or tearing of tendons or muscle fibers.

subarachnoid:	The fluid-filled space between the arachnoid and the pia mater.
subcutaneous:	Under the skin.
subcutaneous emphysema:	Air bubbles beneath the skin.
subdural:	Below the **dura mater**.
subungual:	Beneath a fingernail or toenail.
sucking chest wound:	See **open pneumothorax**.
superior:	Above in relation to something.
superior vena cava:	The large vein that carrys blood from the head, neck, upper limbs, and thorax to the heart.
supine:	Positioned with the face up.
syncope:	Temporary loss of consciousness; fainting.
synovial fluid:	Clear lubricating fluid secreted by the membranes lining joints and tendons.
systolic pressure:	The maximum blood pressure exerted by the heart during contraction; also called systole.

T

tachycardia:	An abnormally rapid heart rate.
talofibular ligament:	The ligament that connects the talus to the fibula.
talus:	The highest of the tarsal bones in the ankle; the ankle bone.
tendinitis:	Inflammation of a tendon.
tendon:	Connective tissue holding muscle to bone.
tension pneumothorax:	The condition caused by a buildup of air in the pleural space that collapses the injured lung and exerts pressure on the uninjured lung and the heart.
testis:	The gland in the male reproductive system where sperm is produced.
thermoregulation:	Regulation of body core temperature.
thoracic vertebrae:	The twelve vertebrae between the cervical vertebrae and the lumbar vertebrae with ribs attached on either side.
thorax:	Chest cavity.
TIA:	See **transient ischemic attack.**
tibia:	The large lower leg bone; shinbone.
tibiofibular ligament:	The ligament that holds together the tibia and fibula.
tinnitus:	Ringing or buzzing in the ears.
torsion of the testis:	The painful twisting of the testis on the spermatic cord.
toxic shock syndrome (TSS):	Uncommon infection caused by the bacterium *Staphylococcus aureus*.

trachea:	Large membranous tube extending from the larynx to the bronchial tubes; windpipe.
transient ischemic attack (TIA):	A temporary stroke caused by insufficient blood supply to the brain, with signs and symptoms lasting less than twenty-four hours.
transverse fracture:	A fracture in which the break extends horizontally across the bone.
triage:	A sorting of patients to determine the order of treatment and transport.
tricuspid valve:	The valve located between the right atrium and the right ventricle of the heart.
tularemia:	An epidemic disease caused by a bacteria transmitted by tick bites.
tumor:	A swelling, growth, or enlargement.
tx:	Shorthand for treatment.
tympanic membrane:	The membrane of the middle ear that vibrates in response to sound waves; the eardrum.

U

ulcer:	An open sore or lesion on skin or mucous membranes caused by a break in the skin that fails to heal.
ulna:	The thinner, longer lower arm bone.
umbilical cord:	A cord connecting the fetus to the placenta consisting of two arteries and one vein.
ureter:	The tube that connects the kidney to the bladder.
urethra:	The duct from which urine is conveyed from the bladder out of the body.
urethritis:	Inflammation of the urethra.
URI:	For *Upper Respiratory Infection.*
urinary tract infection (UTI):	Infection of the urethra, bladder, and/or ureters.
urticaria:	A rash of itchy welts, caused usually by an allergic reaction; hives.
urushiol:	A resinous oil responsible for the irritant properties of poison ivy, poison oak, and poison sumac.
uterus:	The organ of the female reproductive system in which offspring are conceived.
UTI:	See **urinary tract infection.**
UV:	For *ultraviolet light.*
UVA:	For *ultraviolet A.*
UVB:	For *ultraviolet B.*

V

vagina:	The muscular tube leading from the external genitals to the uterus; the birth canal.
Valsalva maneuver:	Forced exhalation with a closed mouth, nose, and glottis that causes equalization of the ears and the pulse to slow down.

vasoconstriction: A narrowing of blood vessels.

vasodilation: A widening of blood vessels.

vasogenic: Originating in the blood vessels.

vein: A vessel that carries blood toward the heart.

ventricle: The main lower chamber of each half of the heart.

ventricular fibrillation (v-fib): Rapid, uncoordinated, quivering of muscle fibers in the ventricles of the heart possibly leading to cardiac arrest.

ventricular tachycardia: A fast heartbeat that originates in one of the ventricles of the heart.

vertigo: Dizziness caused by an equilibium disturbance.

vestibular system: The middle part of the inner ear that helps determine balance and orientation.

v-fib: See **ventricular fibrillation**.

virus: A microorganism that depends on the cells of another organism as a host for replication.

visceral pleura: The portion of the pleura in which the lungs are surrounded.

vitreous humor: Clear fluid with which the eyeball is filled.

W

WFR: Wilderness First Responder.

X

xiphoid process: The cartilage protuberance at the lower end of the sternum.

Improvised Litters

In the dire situation where a patient needs to be moved or evacuated, it is best to obtain help. However, a situation might arise where a victim needs to be moved without assistance from Search and Rescue teams.

Carries

It is possible to carry a victim out using one or two people depending on how many people are available and what material is available.

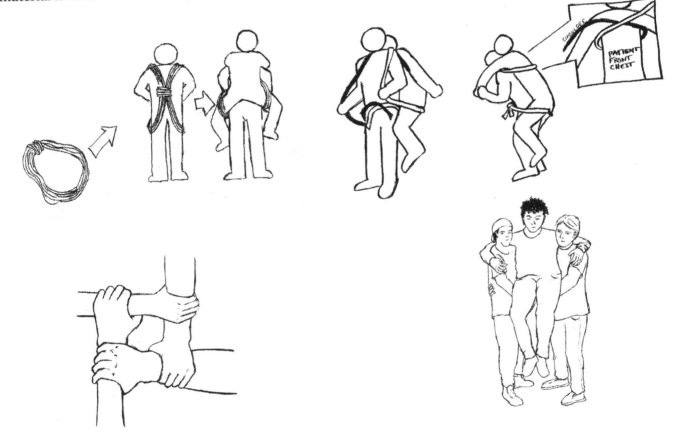

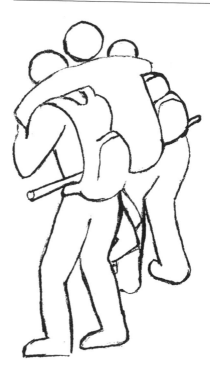

If a litter needs to be created one can be improvised from many different types of objects. Improvisation is the key word. Most flat-surface objects of suitable size can be used as a litter. Such objects include boards, benches, ladders, cots, and poles. If possible, these objects should be padded. Litters can be created by using blankets, ponchos, tents, jackets, shirts, sacks, and bags. Poles can be improvised from s branches, tent poles, skis, and other similar items. If poles cannot be found, a large item, such as a blanket, can be rolled from both sides toward the center. Then the rolls can be used to obtain a firm grip to carry the victim. There are literally dozens of ways that people have come up with to create improvised litters. These are a few of them.

Blanket Litter

You can very quickly create improvised litters using a blanket and two poles. Lay the blanket out flat on the ground, and lay your poles lengthwise across it as shown. Fold one end of the blanket over the first pole. Fold the remaining edge over the second pole. It's really simple but it is prone to slipping over time. This may need readjusting occasionally, but it's an effective improvised litter.

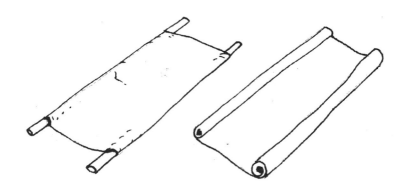

Jacket Litter

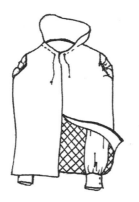

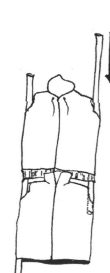

If you have at least two jackets or durable long sleeve shirts available, you can easily fashion improvised litters. This is one of the simplest methods of improvised litters, and is very reliable – as long as the jackets are made of a strong material. Fashion improvised litter poles. Button and/or zip two or three jackets. Turn them inside out with their sleeves remaining on the inside. Pass your poles through the sleeves of the jackets.

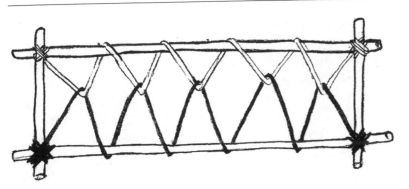

Rope Litters

There are literally dozens of kinds of rope litters. The most important criteria is that they are stable so that the patient is not injured and that they can be created quickly with minimal material.

SOAP NOTE

SUBJECTIVE

OBJECTIVE

LOR:
HR:
RR:
SCTM:
BP:
Pulse:
Temperature: Symptoms:
Allergies:
Medications:
Past medical history:
Last meal:
Events:

ASSESSMENT

PLAN

Wilderness Nutrition

Having a general background in nutrition can have a profound effect on the wilderness experience. As the health provider in the wilderness it is integral that you become aware of the many issues surrounding proper nutrition. By using nutritional skills you can help people have the most enjoyable wilderness experience possible. With proper nutrition it is possible to be full of energy through even the most extreme conditions.

This appendix will give you a basic understanding of nutrition to help you in skills in proper nutritional preparation during the outdoor experience.

The most important lesson that you should learn is that during intense wilderness activities you must hydrate adequately and you must eat a sufficient number of calories for energy, usually as carbohydrates.

The Macro Nutrients

Water

Adequate hydration is the most essential nutritional need during a wilderness activity. Water is needed for all metabolic processes in the body and without an adequate supply you can simply not function.

There are several sources of hydration besides just drinking water such as from the foods you eat and the water produced during metabolism of carbohydrates.

Certain foods, like juicy fruits and vegetables, keep us more hydrated than others. So to maximize hydration it is good if you can eat more of these types of foods. In the backcountry these types of foods are usually more difficult to bring due to their weight, but might be worth the extra weight.

Consuming sufficient electrolytes with your water has recently become a much larger concern. Usually in the backcountry or at home you get a sufficient supply of electrolytes from the food you are eating. When you eat your recommended calories then you really should not have to worry too much about your electrolytes.

But if you find yourself going through a large amount of water or sweating abnormally then you could also not be getting enough of the electrolytes that you need. It is then time to think about an electrolytic supplement either through a sport drink or a commercially prepared product such as a concentrated liquid trace mineral supplement that can be added to you water. This will provide all of the electrolytes that you might have lost.

The amount of water you need a day varies tremendously by how much activity you do, the environmental conditions, and the amount of water in your foods. A good minimum amount of water for a sedentary person is about 2 liters a day. This estimate comes from an approximate requirement of 1 ml of water for every 1 kcal of energy consumed.

Therefore, on a trek in the backcountry you may have to drink as much as 5-6 liters to meet your requirements. Drink water before you become thirsty to make sure that you do not become dehydrated.

A good test to see if you are getting enough water is to ensure that your urine output is plentiful and pale yellow. Be aware that some vitamins such as riboflavin can also affect the color and reliability of this test. Symptoms of dehydration start with about a 1% loss in body weight.

Carbohydrates and Energy

Carbohydrates are the preferred source of energy for our bodies. This energy is used for all types of reactions in the body from movement and thermogenesis to enzymatic reactions and digestion.

We need a certain amount of energy to provide for our daily needs. Exercise or being in extreme conditions can influence this level. Carbohydrates are more easily and quickly broken down than fat and protein into glucose, which is the starting step in energy production.

Carbohydrates are the main source of energy for prolonged high-intensity exercise and exercise in extreme conditions such as high altitude, cold, or heat. A target of 400 g CHO per day or 6-8 g/kg body weight) should be a minimum intake guideline.

```
Signs and Symptoms of Hypoglycemia

- Weak, disoriented, irritable      - Dizziness
- Rapid heart rate                  - Headache
- Pale, cool, clammy skin           - Hunger
- Shallow breathing                 - Blurred Vision

              Give them Sugar!!
```

Carbohydrates are the only source of energy for many parts of the body such as the nervous system including the brain and red blood cells.

Both simple and complex carbohydrates are both used for energy. Simple meaning they are made of only one or two saccharide unites. Complex carbohydrates contain many more even up to 30,000 units. Simple carbohydrates or sugars such as glucose and fructose are readily broken down into energy by the body, while complex carbohydrates are stored for usage over the long term.

```
Tip:
Consuming carbohydrates during high or moderately high
intensity activities can permit a higher work output
```

Glycogen, a complex carbohydrate, is the storage molecule for carbohydrates. One limitation with glycogen is the limited capacity for storage compared to fat. Glycogen stores must be replenished all of the time to ensure a constant supply of glucose for energy.

Complex carbohydrates are found in most of the foods we eat with a large supply in the breads and grain-based foods like rice and pasta. Simple carbohydrates can be found in candy and fruits. There are no specific RDA requirements outlined for the amount of carbs we consume, but it recommended that we eat at least 400 g to replenish our glycogen stores.

The blood glucose level is an important marker for nutritional well-being. There are symptoms for hypoglycemia and hyperglycemia. During wilderness activities you are more likely to encounter some one with low blood sugar. During long intense exercise we will have used all of our blood glucose and muscle and liver glycogen, if this is not replenished then symptoms of hypoglycemia will appear.

It is not a bad idea to carry with you a few pieces of fruit leather, a commercially packaged energy gel pack, or, as a last resort, some hard candy to give to someone if they have symptoms of low blood sugar.

Blood sugar levels are affected differently depending on the type of carbohydrate consumed. The index of how blood sugar level is affected is called the glycemic index. It is important to eat with this index in mind. Foods with a high index, like potatoes, will be metabolized into blood glucose quickly. While those with a low index, like whole grains, will give longer sustained glucose.

Diabetes is the case in which your glucose cannot properly enter your cells causing you to have to high of blood glucose level. Insulin is given to these patients to facilitate glucose entering the cells. In wilderness activities careful watch must be taken that these patients do not become dehydrated due to the hyperglycemia.

Fiber is another essential carbohydrate addition. The fiber in your diet helps you to better maintain your blood glucose levels without dips and spikes. Plants are sources of fiber, so good sources are unprocessed fruits or vegetables. An intake of 25 g of fiber per day may be hard to reach with most backcountry foods but if you can eat this amount, you will be "regular" in the backcountry.

Protein

Recently protein has become a popular topic in nutrition. This section will provide information to help you understand and answer many of the questions regarding proper protein consumption. Protein is not as integral as an energy source as carbohydrates, but it is important for other processes such as the foundation to building muscles, maintaining an active immune system, and facilitating nutrient transportation.

Proteins also are made to act as enzymes and hormones. Also if the conditions require, proteins can be converted and used as energy as a less efficient backup to fat and carbohydrates. Proteins are made of 20 different amino acids of which humans cannot make nine of them. These essential amino acids must be consumed through our diet, which are abundantly found in human food supply.

There are two types of protein in the human diet-- protein from animal sources and protein from plant sources. Animal sources include cheese, milk, meat, poultry, and eggs. Plant sources include soy, nuts, and grains.

In the wilderness setting we often consume protein in a manner that is different than at home. At home we might eat a hamburger or drink a glass of milk to get our protein while in the wilderness grains and cheese might be our main sources of protein. It is important to realize these differences in diet and help explain to others who are used to consuming more visible protein.

The RDA for protein is .8 grams per kilogram of body weight a day. This allows for a comfortable margin of safety as well. This RDA is for the average person people who are regular exercisers could increase their intake. Strength or endurance athletes may want to increase their intake up to 10%.

Protein deficiency, a rare occurrence in the wilderness, has similar symptoms to several other nutritional problems; therefore, you should assess your caloric and fluid intake before concluding that you are lacking in protein. Protein quality is probably a more important consideration than quantity in backcountry considerations. Egg, dairy, peanut and soy proteins are all good sources. There may be some advantage to choosing protein sources high in branch chain amino acids such as whey protein, particularly where undesired weight loss may be a problem (such as at altitude).

Eating too much protein can also be a concern. The extra metabolism of proteins leads to increased nitrogen wastes. These can lead to ammonia build-up in the liver, and place an extra urea burden on the kidneys. These can lead to both liver and kidney damage in the long run. In the short run, the extra protein will require a larger increase in hydration as well as leading to an increased oxidative effect.

Lipids and Fat

Fats are our main source of energy for prolonged mild exercise. In our society we have a mild fear of eating too much fat, and for good reason. Most people eat more fat that the daily recommended dose, which should be from 20% to 35% of our total calories depending on activity level. This fear though should not prevent people from the benefits of fat consumption in the wilderness. Fat provides twice as many calories per gram compared to both carbohydrates and proteins. Fat can also be stored in a more compact manner for use over the long term.

The two main types of fats are saturated and unsaturated fatty acids, which differ in numbers of double bonds between their carbon atoms. Just as with proteins there are fats that we cannot make, but are essential for our bodies. Therefore, we must eat a variety of both types. It is also known however that saturated fatty acids have been linked to increased heart disease. For this reason, it is recommended that we eat less than 10% of our calories from saturated fatty acids.

It is also better to get our fats from natural sources, because processed fats tend to be more prone to oxidation. Heat, air and light, which are used in the processing, tend to contribute to this oxidation. Another undesired byproduct of fat processing is trans fatty acids. These particularly bad plaque causing foods should be avoided, check the food label.

Natural sources for fats include nuts and seeds, such as sunflower seeds, pumpkin seeds and walnuts.

During low intensity exercise we mainly use fat as our source of energy and not carbohydrates. When the intensity of the exercise increases the amount of the amount of carbohydrates being used increases.

Some participants will be used to eating less or perhaps more fat than they will during the wilderness activity. Adjusting to this change could be difficult for them for both psychological and gastrointestinal reasons. It is always best to gradually adapt to or avoid abrupt dietary changes.

Index

Altitude Illness - specific diseases associated, rate of ascent is key
  ~~Altitude~~ - usually ↑ 6,000 ft. is where illness occurs
  - ascending too quickly doesn't allow the pressure in your body
    to adjust quick enough compared to atm. pressure
  - the higher you ascend the slower you need to ascend it
  - breathing rate increases for maintenance of O_2 levels

Acute Mtn. Sickness (AMS)
  - relatively slow breathing, fluid retention (swelling),
    edema, brain begins to swell, incr. intracranial pressure
  - diagnosis is by symptoms - while at altitude → headache
    plus dizziness, fatigue, lightheadness, nausea, insomnia
      - treat early - rest, fluids, oxygen - descent if necessary
      - gradual ascent is key, acetazolamide is best medicine

High Altitude Cerebral Edema (HACE)
      - untreated AMS, swelling in brain alters you
      - long term permanent brain damage
High Altitude
Pulmonary Edema → - takes 2-4 days to show up.
(HAPE) → - fatigue is obvious, coughing, hard to breathe
      - GAMOW bag used to ~~treat~~ - hyperbaric chamber - sometimes

First Aid Kits - geared towards what you're doing!
    - medication dependent? bring extra w/you
    - Adapt & Improvise if necessary!   think about
    - recognize common diseases in ~~to~~ the area   ← getting
                                        gatorade? K(waterproof
                                                bags
                                            Matches?
Water in Backcountry   batteries?
    - pathogens - giardia (common) + e.coli
    - disinfect: remove/destroy pathogens - purify: remove
    - ~~sterilize~~: ~~destroy~~ all life forms   taste, odor, smell
    treatment methods: heat, filter, use chemicals
        bring to rolling boil - doesn't remove chemicals, taste,
            does remove pathogens
    filtration doesn't remove all pathogens, ~~usually~~ not all viruses
chem. treatment → wait longer for colder water + use higher conc.
household bleach works fine - iodine crystals,
chlorine sol. w/taste neutralizer, irradiation
Wilderness Dentistry - pulpitis (toothache) - tooth knocked out - rinse w/saline +
    - cracks/holes in enamel can be packed w/wax or chewing gum   remove debris
    - treat pain if you can't see anything
    - saving a tooth? Hank's balanced pH solution, milk, saliva

Evacuation Guidelines - foot injuries - lightning - seizures, burns, trauma,
    sepsis - skull fracture - heart attack
    - type of injury? stable? can they walk?

Angina - vessels closing / heart problem
  Nitroglycerin - opens veins / arteries
  If rest doesn't relieve pain, GTFO - get to hospital
  congestive — give nitro, O₂ , aspirin
  Heart Failure - people who have this don't go to backcountry worry
    -sickly, cough a lot

    Pneumonia - inflammation in lungs (alveoli) usually w/body infection
      I let them cough + expel : symptoms: shortness of breath, chills, fever,
      hydrate, O₂, antibiotics   chest pain, incr. sputum, productive cough

  Chronic Obstructive Pulmonary Disease (COPD) - very hard to breathe

  Asthma - airway reacts to irritants, narrowing + spasms of airway,
  lots of mucous production, wheezing
    -help patient calm down / relax, epipen if so severe patient can't breathe

law of the wilderness   unconscious, impaired judgment
  contract - written, oral, implied - need permission
    if you offer help + they say yes, you are obligated to stop + stay
    unless you need to leave to get help
  TORT LAW - involves wrongs to people or property
  ⌐Negligence - 1) duty of care 2) failure to perform that duty 3) a loss or injury
      ⌐ that was, 4) caused or contributed to by that failure
      ⌐ exacerbated injury by not acting

Musculoskeletal - consider mechanism of injury - is scene safe?
- ask for both sides range of motion, compare to uninjured side
- if patient can self rescue - that is best

RICES - rest, ice, compression, elevation, stabilization

Tendonitis - injury of overuse, inflammation of a tendon
tendon - connects muscle to bone
ligament - bone to bone

Sprains - injuries to ligaments, pulled/stretched, don't weight
usually more swelling + bruising then a broken bone
- heals in 1-2 wks

Second degree - ligaments partially torn, heals in ~6 wks

Third degree - ligament completely torn, ruptured, joint immovable

Strains - pulled tendons

Made in the USA
San Bernardino, CA
11 June 2015